INFERTIL

The Last Se

INFERTILITY
THE LAST SECRET

*What happens
when you want to have a baby*

Anna McGrail

BLOOMSBURY

First published in Great Britain 1999
Bloomsbury Publishing Plc, 38 Soho Square, London W1V 5DF

Copyright © 1999 by Anna McGrail

Illustrations. Copyright © 1999 by Kate Simunek

The moral right of the author has been asserted

A CIP catalogue record for this book
is available from the British Library

ISBN 0 7475 4396 8

10 9 8 7 6 5 4 3 2 1

Typeset by Hewer Text Ltd, Edinburgh
Printed in Great Britain by Clays Limited, St Ives plc

Contents

Acknowledgements

Many, many people helped me with the writing of this book, and they are mainly women who were at various stages in their journey towards a family. I have been constantly astonished at their honesty in sharing what were sometimes their most painful thoughts and their deepest fears. Often the partners of those women were willing to talk to me as well, and I am pleased to include their comments here because, even though women are the focus of many fertility treatments, that doesn't mean the man is not involved. Wanting a baby is something a couple decide on together, not in isolation.

Some people chose to have their experiences included anonymously, either because even their closest friends and family did not know what they were going or had gone through, or to protect the privacy of their child or children as they grew. Others felt that they were proud of what they had done and were happy to have their names set down in print, and yet others simply wanted to use their own names in a spirit of honesty, with a conviction that the more people are able to be open about infertility and the issues it raises, the easier it will be for other couples in the future.

Many support organisations spent time providing me with details of what they could offer, and many nurses, doctors and consultants took the trouble to answer my phone calls and letters about technical and medical details in a spirit of generosity and goodwill. Thanks also to Jane Moody for providing invaluable information about references.

But for all those who chose to share with me so openly and honestly how you felt, especially those who did not yet know how their journey would end, this book is for you.

Introduction

Most of us take it for granted that we will be able to have children. What is more, we usually assume that it will be at a time of our choosing. We take sensible birth control precautions and concentrate on our careers, or we get married young and hope to start a family straightaway, or we meet a new partner later in life and decide we would like children together even if one of us already has children. Sometimes we make a definite decision to start 'trying for a family'. Quite often we don't make such a definite commitment but simply slide towards it, hoping it will just happen in its own time. When it doesn't happen, and the months tick by and it still doesn't happen, the sense of failure, frustration and anguish can become overwhelming.

There have always been couples unable to have children. For the greater part of human history, such couples had only two alternatives: they could adopt a child, or they could remain childless. Within the last couple of decades, advances in reproductive technology have altered all that. Techniques such as in vitro fertilisation (IVF) offer hope to couples who could not otherwise have had their own genetic offspring. In addition, there are many couples who have already had one child but have what is often called 'secondary' infertility, and there are couples who have few problems conceiving but are then unable to carry a pregnancy to term. In both of these circumstances, too, medical advances now offer hope.

Of course, not everyone will want to pursue all the options that technological progress opens up to them. For various moral, religious or personal reasons, some couples will decide not to undergo treatment that requires the use of donated material – sperm or eggs – or to use techniques involving the freezing of embryos, for example. Others will not rest until they have exhausted every avenue that science can provide. Just how far to go in our quest for children is a decision every couple has to make, but it's a decision that becomes increasingly difficult once we step on to the road and begin fertility treatment. This is not only because we're soon lost in a world of acronyms (ICSI, SUZI, GIFT, IVF and so on), but also because the impression we quite often get is that medical experts consider infertility a 'problem' that can usually be solved, no matter what the cost. For most couples, this is not the case. Indeed, provision for fertility treatment through the National Health Service varies enormously between health authorities – many couples will be offered very little help at all – and the costs of private treatment put it beyond the means of many. In addition, even for couples who can afford it, high-tech solutions offer no guarantees: many couples, at the end of their cycles of treatment, will still not have a baby.

The feelings surrounding the experience of infertility are often strong and sometimes destructive: rage, anger, sadness, despair, isolation. This is in contrast to the cool and rational world of timed injections and precise quantities of drugs which pervade the factsheets and information leaflets we scour through looking for answers. When we have feelings this strong, who can we share them with? We may see our friends conceiving easily, often 'by accident', and even in a spirit of complaint about the children they have already got. Our parents may drop dark hints about becoming (or not becoming) grandparents. Our brothers and sisters may start families of their own and we wonder if we are to be forever cast in the role of aunt or uncle. As for colleagues at work, if they're not on maternity leave of their own we often assume they will be far more interested in the latest project in the office than in our cherished hopes for a family. And besides, if you've been branded a failure for your inability to conceive – and the language of infertility treatment is littered with phrases such as failed treatment cycles, inefficient ovulation, poor sperm counts, incompetent cervix – who do you want to admit that to?

Perhaps that is why, even though approximately one in six couples of childbearing age will seek medical help in conceiving, it is one of the least talked about topics of our age. Infertility really does seem to be 'the last secret'. It's partly because couples feel that they have no one to turn to who will understand what they're going through, and partly because admitting their failure would seem like accepting defeat, and partly because their emotions are so strong that they don't always know how to explain them to anyone else. Besides, there's always next month. . . . Who knows? We might just be successful then, and our 'problem' will magically disappear. It's very hard not to be taken over by that hope.

Another aspect that makes it very hard to share how you feel about using assisted conception techniques is the enormous public debate that they have generated in the media. Journalists often focus on the extreme cases, since these stories sell newspapers. The situation of Diane Blood, whose late husband had not been able to give written consent to the use of his sperm for artificial insemination, generated widespread coverage. The successful experiments with sheep at the Roslin Institute brought cloning to the top of the list of ethical concerns and raised fears about genetic meddling just at a time when pre-implantation genetic diagnosis was beginning to offer couples a greater chance of ensuring that their children were free of inherited disease. A mother who is over sixty is not the norm. People who have seven or eight babies are very few and far between. But they make great front pages. There is no news value in a couple in their late thirties, who have no children and have tried for many long and difficult years, and yet still don't manage to conceive.

Balancing progress and public concern is never easy, and couples who want to make use of cutting-edge treatments may find themselves under attack, often from those less well informed than themselves. People who have never needed to use IVF, for example, may still voice strong opinions, often quite hurtful ones, about whether this treatment is morally, ethically or socially acceptable. Can you risk telling someone you are starting treatment if there's a possibility that they'll just laugh and tell you to be careful not to end up with seven all at once? If they are busy coping with children of their own, how can they understand your desperate desire to have just one? And if they don't have children, how can you share your feelings without appearing to disparage their life choice?

Because of this isolation, the actual experiences of infertile couples have been placed at the centre of this book. Set in the context of factual information about investigations, tests and treatment options, these couples tell what it felt like for them, how they made the decisions they did, and how they reacted when things did or did not go as they had expected. My hope is that these first-hand accounts from those who have experienced the pain of infertility will offer you support if you are considering or undergoing treatment yourself. In addition, these accounts from those on the front line of what is increasingly becoming the 'baby business' may give you a better idea of what to expect, and may provide a framework in which you can question the options open to you and make informed choices about your next step – whether this is to move forward with confidence and without misgivings, or to step back from the 'treadmill' of treatment without regret.

This book will also be of value to couples who decide to seek fertility treatment of a specific kind in order to overcome a particular problem. For example, some couples will know they carry certain genes which will make conception and/or pregnancy difficult to carry to a successful outcome. Or perhaps they know that any child they conceive risks being born with an inherited disease such as cystic fibrosis, and may choose to make use of techniques such as IVF which allow for genetic screening of the embryos that are produced. Also, couples where one or both partners has a disability which means that they are unable to conceive naturally may need to use medical help in order to have children. Once they are embarked upon the assisted conception process, they too may find that their emotional, physical and financial stresses echo those of other couples.

There are some things that aren't in this book: for a start, overwhelming quantities of statistics on the success rates of various techniques. These will differ from couple to couple, and although the book gives some general indications of how successful a treatment is likely to be, no one except your own doctors can tell you how successful it is likely to be in your own particular case. Similarly, 'league tables' of treatment centres vary from year to year, and you are advised to ask for this information yourself if you decide to go ahead with a specific form of treatment. New drugs are constantly coming on the market, so no one except your own doctor can give an overview of everything you might be offered and what its side-effects might be in your individual case, though the book does include some information about the disadvantages as well as the benefits of certain generic treatment regimes. Finally, infertility is a medical speciality in which new techniques and experimental treatments are continually being developed. Research into immune factors, for example, seems to offer new hope to many couples, but again, only your own doctor can tell you if the new tests and treatments will be of benefit in your case or, indeed, whether they could be offered to you in the mix of NHS and private treatment currently available in the UK.

However, there are also some things that are in this book that aren't always included in discussions on infertility. One is the acknowledgement that, statistically, techniques such as IVF are much less likely to work than to be successful, and it is within this context that I have given space to the stories of couples who have created their families through surrogacy or adoption. In addition, couples who have needed egg or sperm donation in order to have a child talk here about some of the emotional, ethical, moral and personal dilemmas they considered before making this choice. Also, in recognition of the benefits and consolation that many couples derive from national and local organisations, there is a full list of groups and contacts which can offer you specific information and support on a variety of topics. Finally, in an age in which you can get advice from your mailing list companions in California within a matter of hours, rather than waiting three months for your next appointment with your consultant, there is a full account of what the various online national and international self-help networks can offer you.

Making choices is not always easy, and when it comes to making choices about matters that touch the whole essence of our being, that force us to consider the purpose of our lives and the reasons for our very existence, we may feel that we are being faced with impossible demands, especially when we feel alone in making those choices. It is significant that the Act of Parliament which governs the provision of fertility services in the UK makes it a legal requirement that couples undergoing certain forms of treatment must receive counselling. That in itself is an acknowledgement of the complexity of the decisions you may be required to make and the implications that those decisions carry.

The over-riding aim of this book, therefore, is to help you make, from the information given, and the sometimes contradictory personal stories, a choice that is right for you.

1

Back to Basics

This chapter provides an overview of the mechanics of what we learned through our biology textbooks to call 'human reproduction'. While most of us know the basics (the sperm meets the egg, and so on) the physical processes are summarised here because couples who feel they might be having problems conceiving often need to know in greater detail what is supposed to be going on.

Perhaps one of the most demoralising aspects of infertility is that it forces us to look at our bodies as biological machines. For most of us, our sexuality is an intensely private, closely guarded concern. Where's the romance in learning about the tubes and ducts of our basic plumbing? Where's the passionate spontaneity in charting our hormone levels? Many women feel uncomfortable with the notion that they need to explore their 'secret places'. Many men feel that a need to know more about how their reproductive system works casts aspersions on their masculinity or virility.

It's not fair. It's not pleasant to have your impulses and desires reduced to textbook diagrams, or the glorious mysteries of sex reduced to a discussion of mechanics. We want to conceive our children in transports of delight, not with a manual in one hand and a thermometer in the other.

Nevertheless, both men and women need to know in detail how their bodies work if they are to give themselves the best chance of conceiving, especially if they have begun to suspect that they might have problems doing so. There are many reasons why conception does not occur or an embryo does not implant in any one cycle, so an understanding of the complex mechanisms of the reproductive system is vital in determining whether you have a 'problem' or not. If, later on, you do become involved in tests or treatments for infertility, you will need to know which part of the process might be going wrong and the ways in which it can be put right. It will also give you a greater understanding of some of the tests – why levels of a particular hormone are being checked, for example – and so help you feel more in control at a time when everything seems to be slipping out of your control.

Not everyone will need to read this section. If you are *au fait* with your Day 7 FSH levels, you will know most of what is written here. But some couples start treatments with only the haziest notion of what doctors are testing for and why, and find it too embarrassing to ask. Let's start, therefore, with an overview of our basic anatomy.

FEMALE FERTILITY

Talk of a 'biological clock' is particularly apt when we are thinking of a woman's fertility. During our lives we move through three distinct phases. We begin as a child. We leave our childhood behind when we enter puberty, the slow process through which our bodies grow into full maturity. Throughout this time we become aware of another cyclical process: at approximately monthly intervals our ovaries produce an egg which, if we don't get pregnant, is shed with the prepared lining of the womb during menstruation. We leave this phase behind with the onset of the menopause, when our bodies gradually cease ovulation, our periods stop and we are no longer fertile.

It's how the system works throughout that monthly fertile cycle that we need to understand. While the organs mainly concerned with making babies – the ovaries and the uterus – are inside the body, it's important to remind ourselves of what we can see from the outside because it is here that everything starts.

THE FEMALE GENITALS

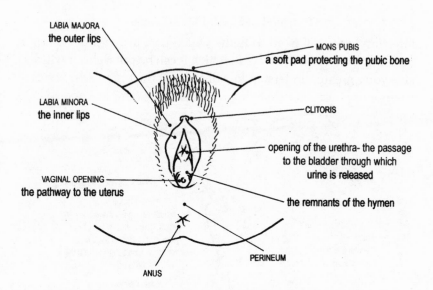

LABIA MAJORA
the outer lips

MONS PUBIS
a soft pad protecting the pubic bone

LABIA MINORA
the inner lips

CLITORIS

opening of the urethra- the passage
to the bladder through which
urine is released

VAGINAL OPENING
the pathway to the uterus

the remnants of the hymen

PERINEUM

ANUS

The basic anatomy

The vulva is the name for a woman's external sex organs. If she looks in a mirror, a woman will see the large, soft lips of the labia majora, which close over the inner lips of her vulva, the labia minora. These inner lips join together at the top of the vulva in the clitoris, a sensitive bud of tissue which is the key to sexual stimulation.

There are two separate openings in the vulva, though not every woman will be aware of this as the urethral opening, through which urine is released, is tiny and often hidden behind the clitoris. More easily visible is the opening to the vagina. Sometimes the vagina is still covered by the hymen, a soft layer of skin. In most women, ordinary physical activities and the use of tampons stretch and break the hymen as we grow, so it is not the reliable test of virginity that legend would have us believe. By the time sexual intercourse first takes place the hymen is often non-existent, but sometimes enough of it remains for intercourse to cause pain to start with.

─────── THE FEMALE REPRODUCTIVE ORGANS ───────

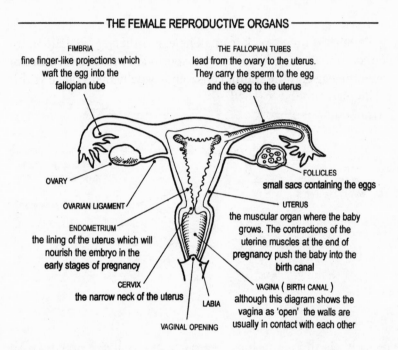

FIMBRIA
fine finger-like projections which waft the egg into the fallopian tube

THE FALLOPIAN TUBES
lead from the ovary to the uterus. They carry the sperm to the egg and the egg to the uterus

OVARY

OVARIAN LIGAMENT

ENDOMETRIUM
the lining of the uterus which will nourish the embryo in the early stages of pregnancy

FOLLICLES
small sacs containing the eggs

UTERUS
the muscular organ where the baby grows. The contractions of the uterine muscles at the end of pregnancy push the baby into the birth canal

CERVIX
the narrow neck of the uterus

LABIA

VAGINAL OPENING

VAGINA (BIRTH CANAL)
although this diagram shows the vagina as 'open' the walls are usually in contact with each other

The vagina is about 7–10 cm long and leads up to the uterus, a pear-shaped muscular organ where any developing baby will be nurtured. If you put your fingers inside your vagina you may be able to feel the cervix, the opening to the uterus, which feels like the tip of your nose. (Sometimes the cervix has a pronounced 'tilt' to it which makes it harder to reach.)

The two ovaries lie one each side of the uterus. About the size of walnuts, they have two main functions: to store, mature and release eggs, the small cells that contain the mother's genetic contribution to any potential child, and to produce hormones. Each ovary contains many follicles, small sacs where the eggs are stored. Approximately every month, hormones influence several follicles to ripen, though generally only one ruptures to release an egg. The release of an egg is called ovulation. Sometimes two or more eggs are released, as happens in the case of non-identical twins (see p. 14).

Once the egg is released, the fimbria, fine hairs at the end of one of the fallopian tubes, pick it up. The egg is then carried along the fallopian tube towards the uterus. If sperm are present, fertilisation – when the egg and the sperm cells join – usually takes place within the fallopian tube.

The uterus has a lining called the endometrium. The purpose of the endometrium is to nourish any newly fertilised egg until the development of the placenta later on in the pregnancy. Each cycle the endometrium thickens, ready to receive a fertilised egg. If the process is working as it should, the endometrium is at its thickest about the time a fertilised egg would reach the uterus, where it will 'implant' itself and pregnancy will begin. If there is no fertilised egg, the endometrium breaks down and is shed from the body at menstruation, when we have a period.

This cyclical renewal and replacement of the endometrium is the most obvious sign of a woman's fertility. Some women breeze through life hardly noticing it; for others, especially during puberty when the system is 'settling in', there may be physical pain or discomfort with each menstruation. Other women find that the varying levels of hormones at each stage of the cycle cause them to feel much better some days than others. In all cases, however, menstruation is a constant reminder of our fertility. The absence of a period may be the first sign that a woman is pregnant; and, of course, for infertile couples, the arrival of a period may bring the crushing realisation that, for yet another cycle, conception has not occurred.

This fertility cycle is influenced by a delicate system of hormones, Each of these 'chemical messengers', which are carried through the bloodstream, has to work in balance with the others. To understand more about a woman's fertility, we therefore need to look beyond the physiology and find out in some detail how these hormones work.

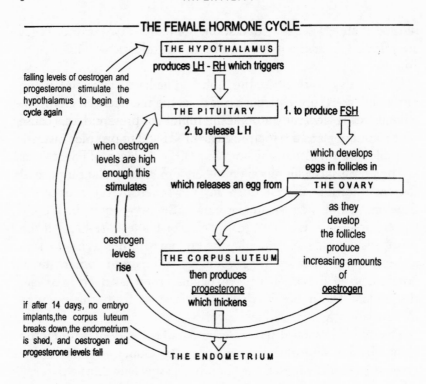

─────────── THE FEMALE HORMONE CYCLE ───────────

THE HYPOTHALAMUS

produces LH - RH which triggers

falling levels of oestrogen and
progesterone stimulate the
hypothalamus to begin the
cycle again

THE PITUITARY   1. to produce FSH

2. to release L H

when oestrogen
levels are high
enough this
stimulates   which releases an egg from   which develops
eggs in follicles in

THE OVARY

as they
develop
the follicles
produce
oestrogen   increasing amounts
levels   of
rise   oestrogen

THE CORPUS LUTEUM

then produces
progesterone
which thickens

if after 14 days, no embryo
implants,the corpus luteum
breaks down,the endometrium
is shed, and oestrogen and
progesterone levels fall

THE ENDOMETRIUM

The dance of the hormones

In each fertility cycle, a woman's hormones work in a series of distinct phases. After each menstruation, the first or 'proliferative' phase of the cycle begins. In this part of the cycle, hormones influence two parallel processes:

- the release of an egg from one of the ovaries
- the thickening of the endometrium in the uterus to receive any fertilised egg

The proliferative phase starts in the brain, where the hypothalamus produces luteinising hormone-releasing hormone (LH-RH). LH-RH triggers a gland called the pituitary in another part of the brain to release follicle-stimulating hormone (FSH). This, as its name suggests, stimulates some of the follicles in the ovary and causes the eggs in those follicles to 'ripen'. As the follicles ripen, they produce increasing amounts of oestrogen. This hormone causes the endometrium to begin to build up.

When levels of oestrogen reach a high enough level in the bloodstream, generally around the middle of the cycle, this causes the pituitary gland to stop producing FSH and to produce instead a sudden surge of luteinising hormone (LH). As levels of FSH fall and LH rise, this causes the most mature follicle in the ovaries to rupture and release its egg. Ovulation usually occurs within 36 hours of the start of this LH surge.

In the second part of the cycle – the 'secretory' or 'luteal' phase, after ovulation – LH causes cells in the ruptured follicle of the ovary to form a functioning gland called the corpus luteum (yellow body). The corpus luteum produces more oestrogen and increasing amounts of the second ovarian hormone, proges-terone. Progesterone stops further follicles from ripening and causes the endometrium to thicken so that it is ready for im-plantation of an embryo. The body then prepares itself for two possible outcomes:

- conception does not occur
- conception does occur and the developing embryo success-fully implants in the endometrium

Sometimes conception does occur, in that the egg and sperm fuse, but the fertilised egg does not then implant successfully (see p. 62), or implantation may happen but the pregnancy is not sustained and the developing embryo is then lost through miscarriage (see p. 194). Each of these possibilities is looked at in more detail in subsequent chapters.

The corpus luteum has a fixed life of about 14 days. If pregnancy does not occur, the corpus luteum begins to degenerate and ceases to produce hormones. Levels of oestrogen and progesterone then fall, and in response the endometrium begins to break down and is shed from the body during menstruation. After menstruation, the cycle begins again.

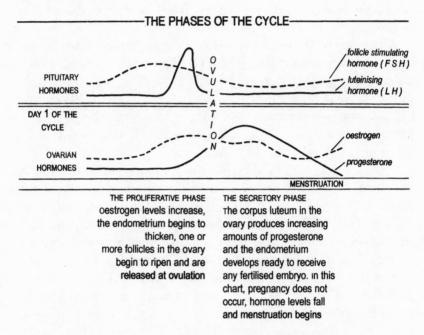

—————————————THE PHASES OF THE CYCLE—————————————

THE PROLIFERATIVE PHASE
oestrogen levels increase, the endometrium begins to thicken, one or more follicles in the ovary begin to ripen and are released at ovulation

THE SECRETORY PHASE
The corpus luteum in the ovary produces increasing amounts of progesterone and the endometrium develops ready to receive any fertilised embryo. In this chart, pregnancy does not occur, hormone levels fall and menstruation begins

If a fertilised egg does implant, the developing tissues in the uterus produce a hormone called human chorionic gonadotrophin (hCG). This maintains the life of the corpus luteum so that levels of oestrogen and progesterone remain high, and as a result the endometrium stays intact and menstruation does not occur.

Although this cycle lasts approximately 28 days, many of us have longer or shorter cycles. It can take varying lengths of time for the oestrogen in the blood to reach a sufficient level to stop the production of FSH and trigger ovulation, so it is the first part of the cycle that is usually longer or shorter. The second part of the cycle tends to vary much less, and for most women the time span between ovulation and the arrival of their period will be about 15 days. Some of us menstruate at regular intervals, no matter what our cycle length, while for others the length of a cycle will vary considerably from one month to the next. At times of stress, too, we may find that our cycle is affected; it is not within our conscious control.

MALE FERTILITY

The most obvious male reproductive organs are the penis and the two testicles behind it; the testicles are contained in a pouch called the scrotum. In the sensitive glans at the tip of the penis can be seen the opening of the urethra. The urethra is the

—————————— THE MALE GENITALS ——————————

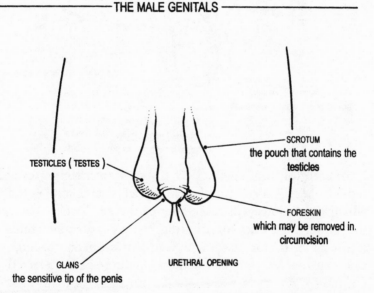

SCROTUM
the pouch that contains the
testicles

TESTICLES (TESTES)

FORESKIN
which may be removed in
circumcision

GLANS
the sensitive tip of the penis

URETHRAL OPENING

passage along which urine is carried to the outside from the bladder, and along which sperm also pass. The glans is usually covered by a foreskin. The foreskin is sometimes removed, for religious, cultural or medical reasons, in the procedure known as circumcision. Whether a man is circumcised or not has no effect on his fertility. In fact, this might be a good place to point out that nothing about the size or appearance of either a woman's vulva or a man's penis has an effect on fertility. It's what goes on inside that counts.

───────────────── THE MALE REPRODUCTIVE ORGANS ─────────────

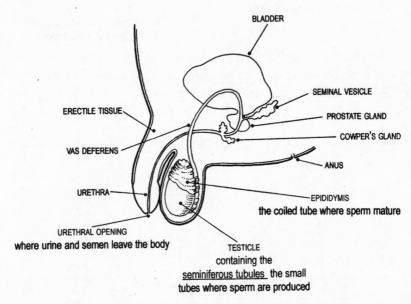

BLADDER

SEMINAL VESICLE

PROSTATE GLAND

ERECTILE TISSUE

COWPER'S GLAND

VAS DEFERENS

ANUS

URETHRA

EPIDIDYMIS
the coiled tube where sperm mature

URETHRAL OPENING
where urine and semen leave the body

TESTICLE
containing the
seminiferous tubules the small
tubes where sperm are produced

   In each of the man's two testicles (sometimes called the testes), there is a system of tightly packed and convoluted tubes which continuously produce sperm, the small cells that contain the father's genetic contribution to any potential child. (The technical term for the male sex cell is spermatozoon, plural spermatozoa, so you may sometimes find sperm referred to in this way.)

   The sperm pass through ducts into the epididymis, a coiled tube about 12 metres long in the upper part of the testicle. When they enter the epididymis, the sperm are not naturally capable of fertilising an egg; it is during their time stored in the epididymis that they mature and become 'motile' – able to move. This process takes about three months.

THE SPERM

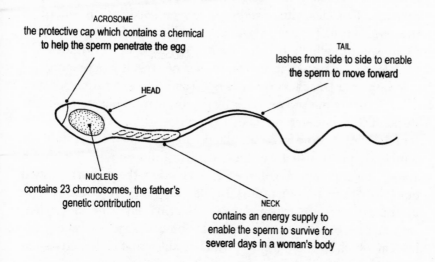

ACROSOME
the protective cap which contains a chemical
to help the sperm penetrate the egg

TAIL
lashes from side to side to enable
the sperm to move forward

HEAD

NUCLEUS
contains 23 chromosomes, the father's
genetic contribution

NECK
contains an energy supply to
enable the sperm to survive for
several days in a woman's body

Sperm develop best at a temperature 2–3°C lower than the rest of the body, which explains why the testes are outside the body. The cremasteric muscles in the scrotum act as a heat-regulating mechanism, and cold temperatures (as well as fear) cause these muscles to draw the testes inside. The Leydig cells in the testes also produce testosterone, the 'male' hormone. While there is no obvious fertility 'cycle' in men, the production of sperm is governed by hormones – not only testosterone but also FSH and LH – which ensure normal sperm development.

Once he reaches puberty and is capable of producing mature sperm, a man is always fertile. His fertility does not ebb and flow in the same way as a woman's through each menstrual cycle. In addition, a man can still produce viable sperm into his nineties: there is no definite end to his reproductive life as there is to a woman's after the menopause, although male fertility does gradually decline.

When a man becomes sexually excited, the blood flow to his penis is increased and it becomes firm – an erection. This allows sexual intercourse to take place, as the penis can then penetrate a woman's vagina. At the same time, the Cowper's glands secrete a fluid which helps to lubricate the urethra ready for sperm to pass through. This clear fluid can often be seen leaking from the tip of the penis during the early stages of sex. (This fluid may also contain some sperm, which is why genital contact, even without full intercourse and ejaculation, can sometimes result in a pregnancy.)

When a man reaches orgasm, a rapid and complex process occurs. The sperm are pushed upwards by rhythmic muscular contractions through the vas deferens. They then mix with secretions from the seminal vesicles and prostate gland to form the seminal fluid, or semen. Semen is usually a thick, whitish fluid, though it varies in colour, consistency and volume. At ejaculation, the semen is pushed out (with quite a momentum) through the urethra. (Although the urethra is the same pathway along which urine leaves the body, when the penis becomes erect the urethra becomes compressed above the level at which sperm can enter, which ensures that urine and semen cannot be released at the same time.)

At each ejaculation, a man will produce on average between 2ml and 5ml of semen. Nature is generous with sperm in comparison to the one egg a woman usually produces in each cycle: each millilitre of semen will contain several million sperm (about 5 per cent of the total volume of the seminal fluid). However, at the end of the journey only one sperm is needed to penetrate the egg for conception to occur.

In the same way that a woman's menstrual cycle is affected by emotional and physical stresses, the reflex mechanisms which control erection and ejaculation are also easily affected by stress, as well as by drugs and alcohol.

CONCEPTION

If that is how the male and the female reproductive systems each work, how do they work together? Leaving aside for the moment the rich tapestry of emotional and physical responses that form a couple's intimate sexual relationship, let's focus on a short summary of how babies are made – again, going back to basics.

This is the 'ideal' scenario. The couple have sexual intercourse, during which the man's semen is deposited near the woman's cervix. The cervix is usually blocked by a fluid called cervical mucus; however, around the time of ovulation, under the influence of increasing amounts of oestrogen, this mucus thins to allow sperm to pass through. If the couple have sex at the right point in the cycle, therefore, the sperm will be able to pass through the cervix, through the uterus and along the fallopian tubes. As the sperm travel, chemical changes mature them further, in a process known as capacitation, which means that they become capable of fertilising an egg.

While this is happening, the woman produces one mature egg from one or other of her ovaries and this is released into the appropriate fallopian tube. Waiting to meet it, or arriving shortly afterwards, are the man's sperm. The moment of conception, when a single sperm penetrates and fertilises the egg, usually takes place in the fallopian tube. The fertilised egg (sometimes called a zygote) then travels down the fallopian tube and into the uterus. There, about nine days after ovulation, it implants into the endometrium, which has been success-fully thickened by the effects of oestrogen and progesterone. The growing embryo is then sustained by hormones from the corpus luteum until the developing placenta can take over and sustain the pregnancy. About nine months after conception, the developing baby is ready to be born.

Boy or girl?

The sex chromosome contained in the egg is always of a type called the X chromosome. The sex chromosome carried by the sperm will be one of two kinds: X or Y. If it is an X, the resulting XX combination created when the egg and the sperm join means the child will be a girl. If the sperm that fertilises the egg carries a Y chromosome, the resulting XY combination will give rise to a boy.

FERTILISATION

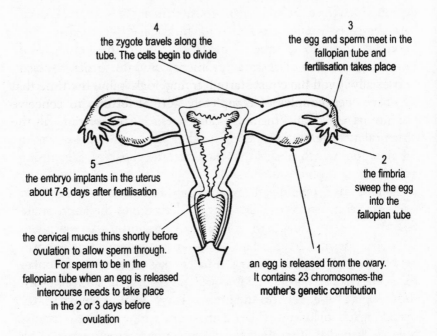

4
the zygote travels along the
tube. The cells begin to divide

3
the egg and sperm meet in the
fallopian tube and
fertilisation takes place

5
the embryo implants in the uterus
about 7-8 days after fertilisation

2
the fimbria
sweep the egg
into the
fallopian tube

the cervical mucus thins shortly before
ovulation to allow sperm through.
For sperm to be in the
fallopian tube when an egg is released
intercourse needs to take place
in the 2 or 3 days before
ovulation

1
an egg is released from the ovary.
It contains 23 chromosomes-the
mother's genetic contribution

Twins or more?

If two eggs are released from the ovaries, they may be
fertilised by two different sperm. The two resulting children
(or triplets if there were three eggs, and so on) will be
genetically different – 'non-identical' – although they may
look alike. As each sperm carries an X or Y chromosome, the
twins could be of different sexes. Identical twins are produced
when the zygote splits just after fertilisation and develops into
two different individuals. Each of these individuals will be
genetically the same, so they will always be of the same sex.
(The only exception is in rare cases of a genetic abnormality
called Turner's syndrome, where one twin is missing a sex
chromosome and develops as a girl even if the other twin is a
boy.)

HOW DO YOU KNOW IF YOU HAVE A PROBLEM?

As the months go by and the woman does not conceive, many couples begin to wonder whether they have what the medical profession would class as a 'problem'. But do remember that, especially if you have just started 'trying' for a baby, the time that it takes even couples of completely normal fertility to conceive varies a great deal. Pregnancy does not occur every time all the ingredients (eggs and sperm) are in the right place at the right time and everything is working as it should. Pregnancy is a matter of chance, or, as some would say, luck. Some couples will be lucky and roll a six on the dice first time; others will still be trying a year later and it doesn't mean that there's anything wrong – it's just bad luck.

How long should it take you to get pregnant?

The chances of getting pregnant in each ovulatory cycle vary according to a wide range of factors, including how often the couple have sex, but perhaps the other most significant factor is that fertility decreases with age.

The chances for conception in each cycle	
If you are aged	Your chances are
20–25	25%
25–30	20%
30–35	15%

After 35, the chances are about 10% for each cycle, and the percentages continue the downward trend with increasing age.

You can see from this chart that human reproduction is relatively inefficient. Even if all systems, physical and hormonal, are working well and intercourse takes place at an appropriate time, you have only a one in four or five chance of achieving pregnancy in each cycle. This means that it will take a couple in their early twenties about five cycles on average to conceive. Women in their early thirties will get pregnant, on average, after nine cycles. But, according to the luck of the draw, one in ten couples without any fertility problems will take more than one year to conceive; one in 20 (5 per cent) will take more than two years, just by chance.

Of course, statistics are just that: generalisations, and in no way individual, so your real chances of conceiving may vary widely. It will usually take longer for older couples, especially for women from 35 onwards. (Unfairly, the man's age is a less significant factor, although some recent studies have suggested that men have a 'biological clock' too.) If you have postponed having children until later in life, it will therefore take you longer to conceive, on average, even if there are no fertility problems.

You can't change your age but this chart may reassure you that the length of time it is taking you to conceive is not abnormal; or it may prompt you into taking further action.

Sex and fertility

The best route to conception is frequent sexual intercourse. If you are having problems with intercourse, this may lead to problems with fertility (because the sperm and the egg don't meet) but does not necessarily mean that you can't conceive. There are all sorts of things that can interfere with intercourse. A woman may find it painful or uncomfortable; so might a man. As a couple, either one or both of you may not feel like sex very often. If you've been happily having intercourse twice a year, this is fine . . . until you want to have a baby.

If a man is unable to gain or sustain an erection, this is known as impotence. There are a variety of contributory medical causes, including diabetes, some prescription drugs such as antidepressants, and some non-prescription drugs. Whatever the cause, if a man is unable to maintain an erection for long enough to ejaculate inside the woman's vagina, this will cause infertility problems for the couple. However, a man who is impotent can still be extremely fertile, in that he is capable of producing sperm which can fertilise an egg. (Conversely, a man who is extremely potent may still turn out to be completely infertile.)

All of these factors can and need to be sorted out well in advance of embarking upon any more intrusive treatment for an 'infertility' problem that may not exist. If these factors affect you, you need to talk to your GP, a counsellor, Relate, or a therapist . . . and each other before doing anything else.

So when should you go to the doctor?

You can see from the figures above that most couples actively trying for a baby will become pregnant within one year. This is why a common definition of 'infertility' is 'the inability to become pregnant after one year of well-timed intercourse'. This is a useful definition because it reminds us that many of the couples considered 'infertile' ('subfertile' might be a better term), do go on to have children – it just takes them longer to conceive than most.

Few GPs will therefore consider that you have a fertility problem, whatever your age, until you have been having regular sexual intercourse (without using any contraception) for at least a year and haven't managed to get pregnant. Only then does it become more likely that there is a real, identifiable reason why you are not conceiving, and this can be investigated.

However, you may feel that waiting for a year is inappropriate if:

- you have conceived before and miscarried
- you are over 30 and feel that time is running out
- you suspect that you might be having problems with ovulation (perhaps because of very long or irregular cycles or painful periods)
- either of you has had a sexually transmitted disease

- you have had abdominal or pelvic surgery (or the man has had surgery in his groin or an injury to his testicles)

All these factors can lessen fertility, so in these circumstances, you are justified in asking your GP to arrange straightforward sperm and ovulation checks after you have been trying for six months. As fertility decreases with age, it generally makes sense to seek help sooner rather than later if you are over 30, since if there is a fertility problem there is less time available to put it right.

KNOWING YOU NEED HELP

There are some situations where a couple will already know that they will need help, often without the need for testing. These circumstances include:

- one of the couple has had treatment for cancer (chemotherapy and radiation can affect fertility in both men and women)
- some women go through a very early menopause (for example, while they are still in their twenties)
- some women will have had their ovaries or uterus removed because of illness (or been born without them)
- a man may have had a vasectomy, perhaps during a relationship with a previous partner
- one of the couple may have a chromosomal condition: Turner's syndrome, for instance, affects women and can mean that she is unable to get pregnant or conceive only with difficulty, while Klinefelter's syndrome affects men and leads to fertility problems

There are also some couples who can't conceive naturally because they can't have intercourse, for example when there is a spinal injury in the male partner. Alison always knew that she and Peter would need fertility treatment since he had severed his spinal cord in an accident.

'We were married before the car crash and until then had always thought that one day we would have children. Practically the first question I asked when he was injured was what the prognosis would be for that. He was then in hospital for six months so we just concentrated on that and him getting better, but it was in the back of our minds all the time. Over the next year or so, we read all the literature and saw someone at Stoke Mandeville [the specialist hospital for paraplegics] who was involved in research into helping couples in our position. We did know we couldn't do it on our own.'

WHAT NEXT?

If you are certain you are having intercourse at the right time (see p. 25) and you have been trying for a baby for long enough to give you cause for concern, you have several options:

- do nothing
- contact one of the support and information groups (see p. 277) which may give you more insight into your particular situation and be able to answer any questions
- embark upon baby-making as a project using only materials you can find at home
- decide to seek medical treatment to help you conceive

Seeking medical advice is a big step for most couples. Making this decision is covered in more detail in Chapter 4.

Some couples decide that under no circumstances would they wish to seek medical treatment, preferring to foster, or adopt, or adjust to the fact that their relationship will not include children. Childlessness can be a positive choice, and no one should feel pressured into thinking they automatically have a 'problem' if they don't have children.

Many couples, however, take a middle route, at least for a while, to see if they can 'give nature time to work' and improve their chances of getting pregnant on their own. It is these self-help solutions we look at in Chapter 2. Even those couples who do decide to seek medical advice may find them useful, as the wait for treatment can be a long one and anything you can do to maximise your chances in the meantime may be worth considering.

2

Self-help

There are many advantages to making sure that you are in general good health, as this will help your body to provide the optimum conditions for conception and establishing a subsequent pregnancy. There are also many things you can do to make sure you give your unborn child the best possible chance of developing normally.

DOING THE BEST FOR YOUR UNBORN CHILD

Rubella: are you immune?

Most women of childbearing age in the UK will have been vaccinated against the rubella virus in their teens, but this does not necessarily give lifelong immunity. It is therefore advisable to check your immune status with your GP if you are trying to conceive. This can be done with a simple blood test to detect antibodies, and is a step well worth taking. If a developing foetus is exposed to the virus, especially in the first 12 weeks of pregnancy, serious disabilities, including deafness and blindness, can result.

Vitamins and minerals: are you taking a folic acid supplement?

The Department of Health recommends that all women considering pregnancy should take a supplement of vitamin B and folic acid: both have been shown significantly to reduce the risks of conceiving a child with chromosomal abnormalities such as spina bifida. You can get the recommended dose of folic acid at any chemist's. Green leafy vegetables, especially brussels sprouts and spinach, and some fortified breakfast cereals also contain a good amount of folic acid. Before buying a supplement, read the warning at the end of the following paragraph.

Your daily diet: do you know what you're eating?

Some foods carry tiny risks for pregnant women, and you may like to avoid them when you are trying to conceive. These include soft cheeses, especially those made with unpasteurised milk, which may carry a small risk of listeria infection, which can lead to miscarriage; and liver or foods containing liver, such as patés, as these contain a very high level of vitamin A, which is suspected of causing developmental abnormalities in the foetus. For this reason, it is also worth checking any mineral and vitamin supplement that you are taking. You will find that many vitamin and mineral supplements specifically designed for pregnant women or those trying to conceive do not include vitamin A.

Your working environment: is it hazardous?

If you work in an environment that brings you into contact with industrial chemicals such as lead and arsenic, or many types of paints or varnishes, this can adversely affect fertility. If in doubt, talk to your Health and Safety Officer about the risks. If necessary, can you change jobs while trying for pregnancy?

Medication: does your GP know you're planning a pregnancy?

A variety of prescribed medicines can decrease fertility, so your GP needs to know that you are hoping to start a family if he prescribes you a medicine when you are ill. This is just as important for a man as for a woman, as some prescriptions can affect sperm production or development. Some drugs (both medicinal and recreational) can also affect libido (sexual desire) or potency (the ability to sustain an erection), so can indirectly affect fertility. Talk to your GP if you are on long-term medication, and he or she may be able to prescribe an alternative if the original drug is known to have an effect on fertility.

Smoking: have you given up?

You know that smoking is bad for you, but it affects fertility as well. Smoking by either the man or the woman significantly reduces a couple's chances of conceiving. Men who smoke have lower levels of testosterone. Women who smoke are more likely to have an ectopic pregnancy (see p. 236) and miscarriage.[1] Trying for a family may be the impetus you need to give up.

HEALTH MATTERS IF YOU WANT TO GET PREGNANT

As fertility is a continuum rather than an either/or (fertile/infertile) state, learning to understand what can enhance or lessen our natural fertility is often the first step a couple needs to take. Martha started this way:

'I wanted to make sure I tried everything before going to the doctor. I took care over what I was eating, no alcohol, no caffeine, started exercising, took mineral supplements, and told myself that I was doing all this to get me in the best of health first, not so a baby would appear. And after a few months I felt so much better and on our summer holidays we conceived. I think my body wasn't ready for it before, but then it was.'

There are things that both of you can do to increase your chances of getting pregnant, and quite often they are simply taking care of your general health. Some of the following points may seem obvious, but they are worth checking to make sure you haven't overlooked anything.

Nutrition: are you eating a healthy diet with not too much fat or sugar and plenty of fruit and vegetables?

Good food is essential to provide the nutrients needed for a man to produce healthy sperm and for a woman to produce healthy eggs. A woman whose diet is severely inadequate may find that she stops ovulating, as if nature recognises that her body is not healthy enough to carry a baby safely to term. Anorexia nervosa, for example, with its deliberate starvation and weight loss to a dangerous level, will cause ovulation to cease completely.

While a balanced diet with the right nutrients is all that most of us need to stay fertile, many people believe that taking particular vitamin and mineral supplements can actually increase your chances of conception. (An organisation called Foresight can provide detailed advice on analysing and coordinating your diet to enhance your fertility: for details see p. 279.) However, John Parsons, head of the King's Assisted Conception Unit (at London's King's College Hospital), feels that if a couple have been diagnosed as infertile and are in good health generally, taking vitamin and mineral supplements will actually have a minimal impact on their chances of conception.

Weight: are you severely underweight or overweight?

In men, excess weight affects sperm production. In women, excess weight can lead to high levels of oestrogen which can prevent ovulation. In women who are severely underweight, the endocrine system stops producing the hormones needed for conception. Even fasting for one day can affect hormone levels the following night, so if you are planning to become pregnant this is not the time for drastic dieting. Even if you need to lose some weight, eating regular, healthy meals is still vital.

Alcohol: how much do you drink?

While there is no evidence that alcohol affects conception, it is known that it can affect a developing foetus. Some couples decide to abstain from alcohol completely while they are trying for a baby, while others find that a glass of wine helps them relax. Alcohol is only a problem in excess.

Underpants: does the man wear boxer shorts?

Wearing tight underpants or jeans can raise the temperature of the testes and lower sperm production and healthy development. It's worth a thought.

Exercise: are you staying fit?

Overdoing exercise can affect ovulation. Not doing any at all will make you seriously unfit. Regular exercise will help you maintain fitness and can also help alleviate the effect on the body of the stress which some couples experience when they have difficulties conceiving.

ARE YOU HAVING SEX AT THE 'RIGHT' TIME?

Throughout each ovulatory cycle, a woman will be more fertile on some days than others – in other words, sexual intercourse on those days is more likely to result in a pregnancy. If you don't get pregnant as soon as you thought you would, it may just be that you've been having sex on the days when the chances of conception were poor.

How can you tell when it's the 'right' time?

As we've seen, conception depends on sperm being in the right place at the right time, ready to fertilise the egg at ovulation. The timing of intercourse is therefore crucial for conception. Once released from the follicle in the ovary, the egg has a short lifespan of between 12 and 24 hours. Sperm can live a little longer, for up to five days inside a woman's body. However, for the best chances of sperm being in the fallopian tube when the egg is released, intercourse has to take place about two or three days before ovulation.

It's obvious, therefore, that knowing when ovulation is taking place is a major clue in knowing when to have intercourse. Unless you're a very lucky person with a textbook regular 28-day cycle, and can therefore predict that ovulation is likely to occur mid-cycle, you may never know when it's taking place. Because the corpus luteum has a fixed life of approximately 14 days, the second phase of the cycle tends to vary little in length. The first phase, however, can vary a great deal, not just between individual women but in the same woman from cycle to cycle: sometimes ovulation may take place on Day 12, at other times not until Day 22, for example.

Some women do experience other indications of ovulation, such as pain on one side of the lower abdomen (caused by the ovarian follicle bursting and releasing the egg), breast tenderness or increased sex drive, but these vary widely from one woman to another. Some women find these signs very accurate, while others do not experience them at all or find them of limited help. Luckily, there are other natural changes within a woman's body which can help many women to work out when the 'fertile' days might be within the rhythms of each menstrual cycle. The fertile days are those just before (and possibly, some would argue, a few hours after) ovulation.

The two main natural indicators which a woman can use to develop an awareness of her own fertility patterns are:

- body temperature changes
- cervical mucus changes

In addition, ovulation predictor kits which measure the changing levels of hormones within your body can help you predict the 'best' time for intercourse. You can use as many or as few of these indicators as you like. They don't work equally well for all women, but experimentation can help you find a method that works for you.

Measuring your cycle

In a biological sense, menstruation is the end of the natural cycle. The endometrium breaks down because no fertilised egg has implanted, and this needs to be shed before the uterus and ovaries start preparing for potential pregnancy all over again. However, because the first day of a period is such an easily recognised 'landmark', this is the day we count as 'Day 1' when charting a menstrual cycle. (To be accurate, Day 1 is the first day of fresh, red bleeding, not the brownish discharge we sometimes see a day or two before.) You then count all the days up to, but not including, the first day of the next period. While 28 days is often given as an average, you may find when you begin to chart your cycle that it varies from this.

Temperature changes

The progesterone that is secreted by the corpus luteum after ovulation often raises a woman's basal body temperature (BBT) very slightly, by around $0.2°C$, and keeps it at this higher level until menstruation begins. To see this rise, you need to take your temperature every day and record it on a special chart.

How to make a BBT chart

1. Choose a thermometer. There are special 'fertility' thermometers available which cover a limited range of temperatures at larger magnification, making the small changes easier to read. Use the same thermometer throughout your cycle, as differences in sensitivity can affect your readings.

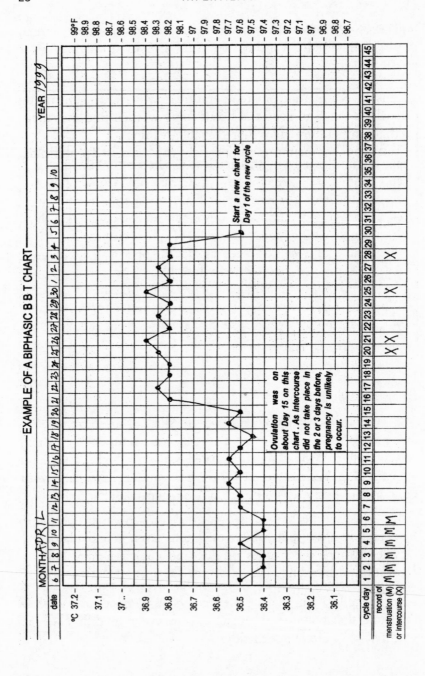

EXAMPLE OF A BIPHASIC B T CHART

MONTH APRIL   YEAR 1999

Ovulation was on about Day 15 on this chart. As intercourse did not take place in the 2 or 3 days before, pregnancy is unlikely to occur.

Start a new chart for Day 1 of the new cycle

2. Decide how you are going to measure your temperature. You can do this orally (by leaving the thermometer in your mouth for five minutes) or internally (via your vagina or rectum, which will take about three minutes). Keep to the same method throughout a cycle as the internal and oral temperatures may vary. The oral route is usually enough to keep track, but some women find that their internal temperature gives more reliable readings.

3. Take your temperature immediately you wake in the morning before doing anything else. Activity will cause a fluctuating rise in temperature which will make your BBT chart harder to interpret.

4. Transfer the temperature reading on to a chart (draw up one of your own or photocopy the blank chart on p. 30.) Start a new chart on Day 1 of your cycle and take your temperature at approximately the same time every morning after that. If your period starts during the day, transfer that morning's temperature reading to Day 1 of a new chart.

5. There is space on the chart for recording when sexual intercourse takes place. This makes it possible (if only with hindsight) to see if it took place close enough to ovulation to give you a chance of conceiving.

For some women, the rise in temperature which occurs just after ovulation is clearly seen between one day and the next. A chart which shows this pattern is called biphasic.

A 'textbook' chart is shown opposite.

Tracking ovulation

Just because you have a period every month or so doesn't necessarily mean that you are ovulating. Even in anovulatory cycles (where the ovaries produce no egg) you may have withdrawal bleeding, caused by the fall in oestrogen levels. Charting can help to show if you are ovulating regularly, irregularly, or not at all.

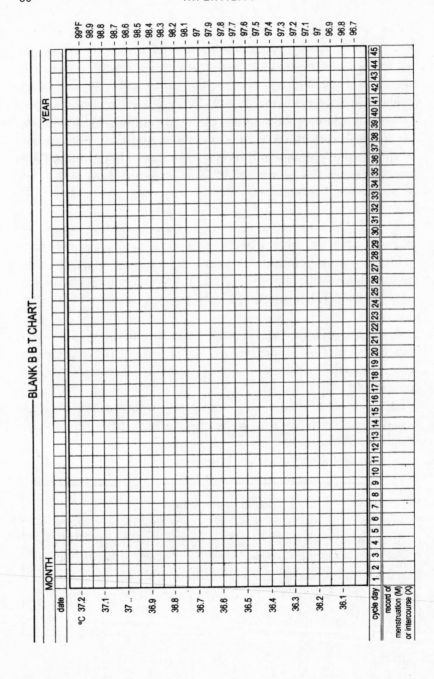

BLANK B B T CHART

Interpreting charts

A few lucky women, whose BBT charts regularly show an easily recognisable rise in temperature, will be reassured that they are probably ovulating. Naturally, not every woman will find her charts so easy to interpret. Sometimes the temperature rises slowly over several days, sometimes in a series of steps. And sometimes any rise at all is hard to pinpoint and yet a woman will still have ovulated. In addition, many things can interfere with the normal pattern: illness, stress, a night on the town, to name but a few.

Cathy found her BBT charts helped her to understand what was going on inside her body.

'I'd always thought it might take me a while to get pregnant as I had very irregular cycles, but that's as much as I'd ever thought about it. After about two years of nothing happening, I got books out of the library and started reading up about it, and started keeping charts, which made me fairly sure I wasn't ovulating every month. That was very helpful. Until then, I never even knew when ovulation was supposed to be.'

Emma is currently keeping BBT charts and finds that they haven't provided the answers she hoped for:

'I thought they would be the answer to everything but they're proving very difficult to work out. I'm not even sure I'm ovulating every month as I don't seem to be having the temperature rise all the books talk about. Also, my cycles have, over the last eight months, varied in length – from 29 days to the last cycle, 43 days. Once I thought I was definitely pregnant . . . only to face the inevitable disappointment. I wish I had a little light that blinks to tell me when I'm ovulating. Wouldn't that make life easy?'

One of the main things to remember about BBT charts is that they are of limited value in helping you to *predict* when ovulation is about to take place. The temperature rise is a response to ovulation, not a signal that it is about to happen. Even if you have intercourse immediately after you see the temperature rise, it may already be too late for the sperm to reach the egg in that cycle.

Nevertheless, keeping a BBT chart may be the first thing your doctor asks you to do if you have any concerns about your fertility, so many couples find themselves keeping them regardless. If you are asked to keep, or decide to keep, a chart, bear in mind that there are advantages, despite the obvious drawbacks.

Advantages of BBT charts

- couples who assumed that ovulation always occurs on Day 14 of a cycle can reassess their estimations of when their most fertile time might be, especially if ovulation generally occurs earlier or much later than this
- charts can show whether you are generally having intercourse near enough to ovulation to maximise your chances of conception, or whether you're simply mistiming sex. This may reassure you that you don't have a problem, for example, if you can see that you've only been having sex too late in the cycle
- BBT charts play a useful role in alerting couples that there might be a problem, and then they can decide what to do about it. Charts which consistently show no temperature rise (anaphasic charts) can indicate that ovulation is not occurring, for example
- if you decide to seek further treatment, a series of charts may also help to convince your GP that intercourse is taking place at the right time even if conception isn't.
- charts can provide a baseline showing a woman's general pattern of fertility which can be of help in determining the best sort of medical treatment if the couple decide to seek further help

Disadvantages of BBT charts

- temperature can be affected by many factors, making the charts hard to interpret.
- they do not predict when ovulation will occur in any one cycle. In a short cycle (of approximately 21 days, for example) ovulation may occur on Day 7. In a longer cycle (of around 35 days), it may not occur until Day 21. For this reason, they can't always help couples to plan the best days to have sex
- they require a great deal of motivation and commitment, as daily temperature-taking can be very restrictive
- they can become a source of panic for couples whose charts show that ovulation is probably occurring and they are having intercourse at the right time month after month . . . but still don't get pregnant. Don't panic after just two or three cycles, however; even for couples of normal fertility, it will take four or five cycles on average to conceive, despite making sure that everything is getting to the right place at the right time. It may simply take you a little longer

Perhaps the single biggest disadvantage of BBT charts is that they remind you every single day that your fertility is not something you can take for granted. This is something Kirsten has found:

'I really don't know how much more of this I can take, and I've been doing charts for six months now. They are a constant heartache.'

Anne remembers how they coloured her whole life:

'The first couple of weeks you fill in all these temperatures and you're full of hope, then you start wondering, and the week before your period is due is just hell. Every time you get a twinge you think your period's starting, every time you go to the loo you worry you'll see blood and you just live in a total panic.'

BBT charts can put a serious strain on your mental health when you do them for too long. Amanda says:

'My GP told me to stop completing them or they would make me psychotic. I'm an obsessive person, and the little lines up and down were just becoming a focus for all my obsessions. I was ovulating! We were having sex! I needed to accept that and move on, and stop reaching for the thermometer first thing every morning.'

Gail, too, stopped doing them after a while, feeling that:

'You get to know your own body. After a few months, they're not telling you anything you don't know already.'

Cervical mucus

The cells lining the cervix produce secretions of mucus continuously. The mucus is mainly designed to block the cervix and keep out bacteria, but its look and feel change under the influence of varying levels of oestrogen and progesterone. Most women are aware of these changes as the mucus appears in the vagina, and can be seen on toilet tissue or when it dries on underwear, but we don't always link the significance of these changes to fertility.

While we are all different and no two women's patterns will ever be exactly the same, there are some general guidelines. In the early part of the cycle, cervical mucus is thick and sticky. It blocks the cervix and makes it very difficult for sperm to get through. Most of us are not even aware of any mucus at this time. As the levels of oestrogen rise, the mucus becomes more fluid, and more of it is produced. A woman may become aware of thinner, white or creamy secretions in her vagina, and a greater sensation of feeling 'damp'. As ovulation approaches, the mucus become even thinner and clear, with a characteristic 'egg-white' appearance. It will stretch if pulled between your fingertips. This is sometimes called 'fertile' mucus because it is only this thin, clear mucus that allows the easy passage of sperm through the cervix. After ovulation, in response to increasing levels of progesterone, the mucus again becomes thicker and more difficult for sperm to penetrate.

Some women combine examination of cervical mucus with noting changes in the position of their cervix. As ovulation approaches, the cervix rises and softens, and the opening widens. After ovulation, it begins to lower and close up again. This is not something everyone will find easy to do, and when it rises it can be more difficult to reach anyway. However, it is one more natural sign you can use to help you become pregnant.

Fertile days

To maximise your chances of pregnancy, have intercourse on the days when clear, slippery mucus is present in your vagina. If you have also recorded several cycles of BBT charts and can see a general pattern in your ovulation, these two factors combined can help you guess which days in your cycle are likely to be the most fertile 'pre-ovulation' days.

While cervical mucus is one of the best natural indicators of fertility, it is not easy for everyone to keep track of it. Some women are uncomfortable about exploring their vagina with their fingertips to note the changes. Some women also find it difficult to distinguish between cervical mucus and the clear fluid secreted during sexual arousal (the purpose of which is to lubricate the vagina to make intercourse easier). While this does not have the 'egg-white' quality of cervical mucus, its presence can be confusing, especially if you're trying to have sex more often around your fertile time. In addition, the presence of semen can cause difficulties in interpreting the texture of cervical mucus.

Ideally, to allow you to note any changes in cervical mucus during the day, intercourse should take place in the evenings. Some experts even recommend having sex only on alternate days to allow you to note changes more accurately. However, restricting sex to every other evening seems unnecessarily lacking in spontaneity and frequency when you most want to get pregnant.

There are several books available which look at BBT charts and patterns of cervical mucus and give detailed information on interpreting them. Often the emphasis of these books is on natural contraception, but they can also be of use to couples who want to know more about recognising when they are most likely to get pregnant.

Ovulation predictor kits

Because sperm can live for some days inside a woman's body, having sex in advance of ovulation is your best bet for getting pregnant, and this is where ovulation predictor kits (OPKs) come in. Ovulation is triggered by a sudden surge of LH (luteinising hormone) within the bloodstream. OPKs work by detecting the appearance of this LH surge, thus signalling to a couple that they are now in the most fertile days of the cycle.

Generally, a woman carries out the test by urinating on to a 'dipstick'; a colour change on the dipstick a few minutes later will identify if levels of LH have begun to rise. Some tests involve collecting your urine in a container and mixing it with the test chemicals. Often the test is carried out first thing in the morning (when levels of hormones are usually at their most concentrated) though some tests suggest the afternoon; it won't make a great deal of difference as long as you do it at the same time each day. A woman will need to test for up to five or ten days in each cycle. Exactly which days will depend on her usual cycle length and regularity. You can stop testing once you see the positive sign, because this indicates that the LH surge has begun. This signals your time of maximum fertility, as most women ovulate between 12 and 36 hours later.

However, Gilli found that her OPK didn't give her enough warning of when ovulation was about to happen.

'For the first few months we'd wait for it to change colour, but it wasn't always possible to schedule in sex within the next twelve hours or so, and I became fairly sure that we were missing ovulation. So then we began the game of trying to predict the predictor kit.'

Karen, too, found that OPKs didn't help her, and after several months of getting false positives, and sometimes no colour changes at all, abandoned them, mainly on the grounds that she was spending a great deal of money for little discernible benefit.

While they are relatively expensive, OPKs can be invaluable for some women, especially those who have cycles of varying length, or whose cervical mucus changes aren't easily detectable.

WHAT ELSE CAN YOU TRY?

Variations on intercourse

There are many (unproven) theories about the right position for intercourse to assure conception, although there is certainly no harm in trying out as many as you like as often as you like.

Some other approaches that couples have tried are:

- the woman lying down for half an hour after sex (so the semen doesn't immediately leak out)
- making sure the woman also has an orgasm (as this helps the sperm to move up into the uterus)
- having sex as often as possible (abstaining from sex can actually decrease sperm quality, so there's no point in 'saving up' for a once-a-month attempt; sperm production seems to work more in accordance with the laws of supply and demand: if more is needed, a man will produce more)

Alternatives

When you are doing everything you can to increase your chances of conception, you may want to consider whether complementary therapies have anything to offer you. Many practitioners, and couples, believe that these therapies can help by restoring the body's own healing mechanisms, and many 'orthodox' medical practitioners are incorporating them into the range of treatments they offer. The main therapies that you might consider looking into are:

- *acupuncture*: this traditional Chinese medical technique is said to help to regulate ovulation and balance hormone levels
- *essential oils*: many aromatherapists believe that extracts of certain plants and flowers can stimulate the endocrine system, balance hormone levels and soothe stress
- *homeopathy*: homeopathic remedies have been recommended for hormonal imbalances and also as a way of preventing miscarriage
- *herbs*: have long been used to treat a variety of infertility problems, ranging from male factor infertility to low progesterone levels
- *reflexology*: reflexologists apply finger pressure to particular points on the soles of the feet with the aim of achieving a therapeutic effect on a particular part of the body; reflexology is said to have beneficial effects on the endocrine system

There are no recipes in this book for magic cures you may like to try. This is for two reasons. First, the absolute essence of any complementary therapy is that it's holistic: treatment takes into account the individual as a whole – their psychological, emotional and spiritual make-up – and doesn't consider one physical symptom or another in isolation. Two women turning up on the same day for help with irregular periods, for example, may be offered very different remedies and treatments. You therefore need to find a qualified practitioner in the therapy you feel would be most appropriate for you. The therapist will discuss with you in detail your history, background and lifestyle, and only then will he or she suggest a way forward.

Secondly, just because some of these therapies have not been fully admitted to be of benefit by every member of the medical profession, that does not mean they cannot be very powerful. Finding a qualified practitioner who can guide you on what treatments could help you, and which would be safe for you, is always a better place to start than leaping in and taking something because you've heard it helped a friend. Details of organisations which can provide you with information about finding an appropriately qualified therapist can be found on p. 280, or you might prefer to ask for a personal recommendation from someone you can trust.

Many stories circulate about the beneficial power of natural remedies, but vital information sometimes gets lost along the grapevine. Eilish, for example, started drinking raspberry leaf tea as she had heard that it had a beneficial effect on fertility. Red raspberry leaves (either in capsules or as a tea) do act as a uterine 'tonic' and have long been used by pregnant women to strengthen and tone the muscles of the uterus, making for an easier labour. However, because they can have such a powerful effect, in early pregnancy they could cause bleeding and prevent the implantation of an embryo. Most herbalists would only ever recommend this tea for the third trimester of pregnancy and then in small amounts, such as one cup a day. Herbs can help, but be cautious and seek advice.

Although Eilish changed her mind about the raspberry leaf tea, she did go on to try other herbs and found that they helped to regulate her cycle and

'just generally, make me feel better about myself. Perhaps one of the most positive benefits was that they made me feel that I was taking an

active, proactive stand about doing something, not just sitting around waiting for something to happen until the next doctor's appointment.'

Not everyone will find these therapies appealing, and not everyone will want to wait the months it will generally take for these treatments to have an effect. For Anne, consideration of alternatives was over in a short time:

'My sister recommended homeopathy and warned me that I might need to give it a few months to work. Well, you have to be patient for all these things to work and I wasn't prepared to be patient. I knew I had a medical problem – I have polycystic ovaries – and I wanted to go straight on to hard drugs to get it solved.'

Probably one of the most beneficial effects of complementary therapies is that they give couples a sense of taking control and doing everything they can to increase their chances of conceiving naturally. There is also no doubt that the relaxing and soothing effects of many of the therapies increase your sense of wellbeing and improve your general health at a time when this is being worn down by the stress of worrying whether you're going to conceive this month.

BE WARY OF MIRACLES

It's almost guaranteed that, if you tell anyone you might be having problems conceiving, they will have a miracle story for you. These often have a folklore quality. 'One couple had been trying for ten years and then they switched to a diet containing yak's milk/ tomato seeds/wild yams'. . . . Gail was taken aback by one suggestion.

'Somebody told me to get a dog. They said, "I know somebody who got a dog and was pregnant within a week." Really?'

There are hundreds of individual success stories of how couples eventually conceived, though often it is impossible to determine if conception really did occur because they switched to a diet containing yams or drank more cranberry juice (or less), or whether this was just coincidence.

Amanda, who admits to having been seduced by some of the miracle stories herself, has a word of warning, however:

'If you've been told by your doctor that there's no obvious reason why you aren't conceiving, then I think you do have to have an open mind and take charge of some things for yourself, as we did. But you're very vulnerable when you're trying to have a baby. It's easy to fall prey to false hopes that something new will be the magic key that you need, and you just feel more let down when it doesn't work.'

If you want a vast choice of miracle cures, the 'Low-Tech Ways to Help You Conceive' online collection of suggestions (see p. 294 for details) is worth looking at, although you should always check with your GP first if you are considering making radical changes to your diet or lifestyle. Gail, who has come across many 'helpful hints' from online support groups, is sometimes shocked at the risks people take:

'It's one thing being on an aspirin treatment regime under the care of your doctor, it's another thing altogether sitting at home and dosing yourself with it because you've heard it's helped someone else.'

The organisation Foresight (see p. 279) can provide you with information about many ways in which you can safely maximise your chances of conception as a couple by bringing your diet to optimum levels, balancing the minerals in your body and eliminating toxins, and this is something you may like to try. As Amanda says, it does you no harm to try to take control by doing something positive; it's when hoping for a miracle begins to take control of you that your stress levels, far from dissipating, will build.

STRESS

Of all the factors up for discussion when trying to get pregnant, the topic of 'stress' probably causes the most stress. Some days you may feel that if you hear just one more person telling you to 'Relax, enjoy yourselves, stop worrying, have a holiday' – whether this is a friend, a relative or your GP – your stress levels will go through the roof. Although often difficult to achieve, especially if one or both of you has a demanding job, relaxation can have a major effect on the body; the stories of couples who unexpectedly conceive on holiday are too legion to be ignored, but that is of no help to you if you've already had three holidays this year and the only consequence has been that you've seen a lot of the world but still don't have a baby.

Does stress cause infertility? Or does infertility cause stress? And if stress causes infertility which causes stress . . . how can you ever hope to break free from the vicious circle?

Take a step back for a moment: in many cases of infertility, there is a clearly diagnosable medical reason. And a medical reason such as blocked fallopian tubes or a complete absence of sperm in the semen can't be caused by emotional stress, so stress cannot be the cause of the infertility.

There is no doubt that stress can disrupt the menstrual cycle: hormone levels vary, ovulation may be delayed. And if your periods do become more and more irregular, this will further increase your anxiety. The effect of stress upon sperm development is less certain. Sperm are produced continuously, and it takes three months for a sperm cell to mature, so any stress wouldn't have an immediate and obvious effect anyway, and no study has been able to show a definite correlation between stress levels and reduced sperm counts.

However, there are many cases where, even if the couple is under severe psychological stress, it doesn't seem to have had the slightest detrimental effect on the process of conception. If it did, there would be probably never be any births during wartime, or no babies conceived at times of famine and flood or in conditions of extreme poverty, and we know that this just isn't the case.

Infertility certainly causes stress. Two areas in particular are the source of much tension:

- having sex at the right time
- and if you have, wondering whether it's 'worked' or not

Baby-making sex

The main impact of trying to time sex so that it takes place in those magic pre-ovulation days – whether you're trying to pinpoint these by using charts, noting cervical mucus changes, using OPKs or a combination of all three – is that sex can move from a spontaneous expression of desire to a planned activity scheduled in for an appropriate date, never mind the prevailing emotions. Premeditation and passion rarely mix. Regulating your sexual activity to coincide with a few precious hours in the middle of the month takes away the element of spontaneity completely, as Andrea found:

'All of a sudden our sex life was taken over with charts and thermometers. And let's face it, announcing that your temperature's risen half a degree is hardly the most alluring come-on.'

Richard felt that his partner, Monica, lost all interest in having sex on nights that weren't the 'right' night:

'She seemed to forget that sex was something you did because you enjoyed it. I felt like it was becoming a chore, on a par with doing the ironing.'

For Gilli,

'Our sex life became so focused on producing a baby that it became almost regimented.'

Jayne also found that charting her temperature 'played havoc' with her love life:

'Temperature charts? They should be banned. They aren't accurate and the minute your temperature goes up you think, that's it, we must do it right now or else we'll miss another month. There were big rows during this time, too, because sometimes Mark would forget that it was my most fertile time and I'd get angry and think he didn't care. Many times we both felt as though we had to force ourselves and this took the passion right out of it.'

Gilli also felt that

'The feelings between us as a couple were often forgotten. Arguments sprang out of my determination to get the timing right, and Adam's not being "all right on the night", as it were.'

Sadly, the things we do to give ourselves the best chance of conceiving may simply introduce another source of stress. And when you are under stress, that can affect your sexuality. You may not feel like it on the 'right' night. Pressure to perform can cause reluctance in both partners, or even impotence or premature ejaculation in some men, therefore adding more stress to what is already a tense situation. Linda says,

'Interestingly, the two times I have conceived have been when my husband had a couple of weeks off work (once in the summer, once around Easter) and his stress level was significantly reduced. It's always the woman who's supposed to get stressed. Why is it men are never told to relax?'

Knowing when the 'right' time is can in itself become a stress factor if, for whatever reason, you have to miss the opportunity that cycle. If your work demands that you travel, or one of you is away visiting relatives, it is easy for frustrations to emerge. And there are unavoidable pressures: Sophie, who was using an OPK, says,

'I saw the colour change one morning, and Stephen arranged to come home early that night. Then during the day we got the news that one of his closest friends had died. We did make love that night, even though neither of us felt much like it. I'm not surprised I didn't become pregnant that month as nothing felt right.'

And even when you're fairly sure you have managed to have sex at the right time, you've still got to wait to find out if this is going to be the month.

AM I PREGNANT?
WELCOME TO THE LAND OF OBSESSION

No one who hasn't experienced them can ever begin to understand those feelings that you get late in the cycle when you might be pregnant. Your temperature hasn't dropped yet, there is definite tenderness in your breasts, and didn't you feel just a tiny bit nauseous when you opened the packed of cereal this morning? Or you might not be.

Barbara admits that she got very little work done in the office on those days because she was 'obsessing like mad', and it is difficult to turn your mind to paperwork when you're sensitised to the minutest changes in your body.

Unfortunately, so many of the bodily changes associated with early pregnancy mirror those symptoms which can arise just before a period starts. Amanda says,

'The thing is, no one can tell you whether these are signs of early pregnancy, or whether your period's about to happen, or whether they're all just psychologically induced. I cannot tell you the amount of times I convinced myself I must be pregnant . . . just for one or two days even . . . only to have every hope

demolished when I saw that familiar faint brown stain on my knickers.'

Gilli, too, talked herself into thinking she was pregnant so many times that her partner told her she should take out shares in the company that produced home pregnancy tests. All negative. Sylvia, who has irregular cycles, also finds the days towards the end of the cycle very hard to deal with.

'My temperature always drops just before my period starts and until that happens, I live in this sort of limbo. It's sometimes a relief when my period does arrive. Of course, it would be much better if I was pregnant, but at least now I know and can stop wondering. Then, of course, you just start all over again . . . .'

Cora notes another strange phenomenon:

'Have you ever noticed how, even if you hold out doing a pregnancy test, and you put it off another day, and then another day, that your period always arrives within hours of you getting the negative result? It's like your body was just waiting for you to admit the fact that you're not pregnant, and then it can go into overdrive with period pains.'

However, the disappointment and depression you feel when a test comes up negative can be doubled when you have a faint positive sign . . . and then it all comes to nothing. Cathy did get a 'maybe' positive home pregnancy test, but her period started a couple of days later.

'I cannot tell you how I felt. Devastated doesn't even come close. But what's even stranger is that I thought my body must be wrong, not the test.'

Home pregnancy tests

Nowadays, tests you can do at home are very sensitive and can pick up the presence of pregnancy hormones in your system even before you have missed a period. However, a positive result does not always mean that your period won't arrive, just as usual, as the pregnancy may miscarry at a very early stage. It is only since pregnancy tests became so sensitive that people have realised how common early miscarriage can be. In the past, these very early losses may not even have been noticed and the woman would never have known she had been pregnant.

Usually women keep many of these feelings to themselves. We put on a calm front, we deal with the paperwork in the office, we distract ourselves by painting the kitchen . . . We usually don't tell our friends the cycle day we've reached and whether this is our longest cycle yet . . . Amanda has figured out the reason she doesn't:

'I get so superstitious about it. If I say the words out loud, "I think I might be pregnant", then I know that my period will immediately start. So I can't say them. Or even think *them.'*

Often the only person to bear the brunt of the emotional fall-out is the woman's partner. Gail admits,

'He says it's like living with a yo-yo.'

Usually, when we are worried about something, we share those worries with a friend, a relative, someone who will understand. But unless someone has experienced these same feelings for themselves it's very hard for them to understand quite how deep they go.

And, of course, one of the main risks in raising the topic of being worried that you might have a problem getting pregnant is that you may well be told – often by someone who has no such problems – that the problem either doesn't exist ('You've got plenty of time yet . . .') or you're making it worse by worrying about it ('Relax . . .').

RELAX?

Sunita, who has been trying for a baby for a year, says,

'I'm under enough stress already without being told to relax and forget about it. I worry now that I'm worrying too much. But how can I stop? I do have something to worry about.'

Similarly, Amanda feels:

'I think about having a child every second of every day. I can't stop "trying too hard" like everyone tells me, because if I don't try it may never happen. People who say things like that really just don't understand.'

Given all this, is it possible to 'forget about it all'? How can we 'relax'? There is one thing which may help. No study has ever been able to show some mysterious endocrinal link between not getting pregnant and worrying about not getting pregnant. Worrying about whether you are going to conceive won't stop you conceiving. If you are therefore beginning to think that the reason you are not conceiving is more than just 'bad luck', perhaps now is the time to visit your GP and find out.

IS IT TIME TO SEEK HELP?

Of course, the moment that you decided to do anything at all about increasing your chances of conception was the moment you made your commitment to wanting to get pregnant. Deirdre was aware of this:

'We were making the very real choice of trying for a baby. I began taking my temperature every morning like clockwork, searching for the subtle, magical change that would mean I was ovulating. I think many people would rather just "let it happen" than commit themselves to this sort of decision.'

I certainly think that most of us would rather just 'let it happen' than make a public statement that you want to become pregnant; which is what going to your GP ultimately comes down to.

Performance anxiety

Some men fear that deciding to seek treatment for a fertility problem will lead people to believe that they have an impotence problem. Thankfully, this attitude is gradually changing as more and more people realise that the two are not necessarily linked. A man could be extremely potent and ejaculate copiously several times a day, yet still not be producing any sperm. This is what tests are designed to find out – not to explore his sexual technique.

If you have been keeping temperature charts for a while, there may come a point where they are simply too much to bear. Helen's period has just arrived – again – and she has booked an appointment with her GP.

'It's devastating. Right now, it's just devastating and I can't stand this any more. I only know that next month can't get here fast enough and I'm wishing my life away, and in the meantime I've got to do something. I can't go on like this.'

Cathy, on the other hand, despite a year of 'trying', has decided not to go to her GP yet.

'I'm so confused and feel guilty for being ambivalent. I read about all the things that fertility drugs can do to your body and think about all the complications of having surgery. . . . Can I really go through all that emotional and physical pain to be a mother?'

Gina, on the other hand, has asked herself the same questions and decided that she doesn't want to delay any longer.

'If there is something wrong, I want to find out about it. I don't want to go through this month after month not knowing, half hoping. I've been trying to avoid it, clinging on to the idea that it might just happen all by itself, but now we've got to know. And when you go to find out if there is a problem, then you have to be prepared for the fact that there might be a problem, haven't you? That's the awful thing about it.'

What next?

You still have two options:

- letting 'nature take its course', even if this means you may never conceive
- going to see your GP

A common reason for many couples deciding to seek treatment is their awareness of how a woman's fertility naturally declines with age. It actually begins declining soon after the age of 25, though most women can become pregnant well into their forties. Another factor to bear in mind is that the rate of miscarriage and birth defects increases after 35, so if you have been trying for a year, even with all the self-help solutions, and still have not conceived, it may be sensible to go to your GP rather than delaying any longer.

If you have a disability that may cause long-term health problems, you may also decide not to wait too long. Robin and Tracy are both disabled people and, after two years trying for a pregnancy without any luck, decided to consult their GP.

Robin, says,

'Although for many people two years is a relatively short time, we felt that time was of the essence to ensure that we were in as good health as possible.'

There is no right or wrong time to make the first appointment with your GP. It depends on your own feelings as a couple. And there is no doubt that it is a big step. You may worry that:

- it signals to the world that you are a failure because you can't conceive on your own
- there is something seriously wrong with you
- your GP won't take you seriously
- your GP will take you seriously and set you off on a round of treatments and tests that you're not ready for

If you and your partner are both committed to having children and you have genuine cause for concern that there may be a medical reason preventing you conceiving, it is probably the right time to go to your GP. But if you are still uncertain, you may like to consider contacting one of the support groups (see p. 278). Talking through your fears and worries, and your hopes, may help you to get things in perspective before you make your decision.

3

What Might Be the Problem?

This chapter provides information about:

- the possible causes of infertility
- the tests you may be offered to find out exactly what the problem is
- the treatment options which may then be available to you

Individual methods of treatment that may be recommended are discussed in more detail in Chapter 5.

Many couples with infertility problems feel that they quickly become lost in a maze. The material here is intended to help you make decisions at each step of the way so that you don't lose your way.

FIRST STEPS

If you have decided to seek medical help in conceiving, your first port of call is your GP. If he feels you need more specialised treatment, you will be referred to a specialist.

Possible treatment path
decision to consult GP
↓
initial tests and assessment
↓
initial treatment
↓
referral to consultant/fertility clinic for more tests
(either NHS or private)
↓
treatment (NHS or private)

Not everyone has to embark on a lengthy process. For some couples, intervention by their GP will work. However, treatment for infertility can take a long time, with no set finishing date and no guaranteed results.

TOGETHER OR SEPARATELY?

It is preferable that you both go together to the GP as the problem may lie on either side. While the figures quoted in the research differ slightly from study to study, the consensus seems to be that for around 35 per cent of couples the cause will be female problems, and for 35 per cent male problems. The cause will be a combined problem of the couple in around 10 per cent of cases, and in 20 per cent no cause is found.

Going together is the ideal, but in many cases women find it easier if they make the initial appointment. This is because men are still more reluctant in general to seek treatment than women, and of course it is easier just to see your own doctor if you have different GPs. However, if there is a problem, at some stage you will need to be seen together because infertility is a problem you share, not something one of you needs to take all the responsibility for.

Open and honest

At your first visit, the GP will ask about your medical history. If you've ever had a sexually transmitted disease, for example, your doctor will need to know, as it can have a lasting impact on fertility. You will also need to be honest with each other as a couple about any conceptions, whether carried to term or not, in previous relationships, or consider what effect your decision to keep such matters secret may have on any future treatment.

Once you've made the appointment, gather together all the information you can – BBT charts, if you've been keeping them, for example. Look at the list of questions below and check if you've got all the information to hand. Think whether there are any questions you don't want to answer, and consider ways you could let your GP know the facts if you don't want to bring them to the attention of your partner.

Also make a list of questions you want to ask at your first appointment and bring paper and a pen so you can take some notes. If you know exactly what tests your GP is suggesting for you and why, this will help you feel more in control of the process.

QUESTIONS YOUR GP MAY ASK YOU

Your doctor will want to know about a variety of factors that have some bearing on your fertility. This will probably start with the easy stuff – how old you are, what you do for a living, whether you drink or smoke, whether you use medicinal or recreational drugs, how long you've been together, how long you've been trying for a baby – and then move on to more difficult matters. Remember, however, that the doctor is only asking these questions because their answers determine how likely it is that you have a real problem.

For both of you

- have you ever had a sexually transmitted disease?
- have you had previous surgery: for a man, especially in the genito-urinary area; for a woman, especially in the pelvic area (like having your appendix out)?
- do you have diabetes?
- how often do you have sex?

For a man

- have you had mumps after puberty or an infection such as prostatitis?
- did you have a hernia repair as a baby (as this occasionally causes a blockage of the vas deferens)?
- have you had a previous pregnancy with another partner?

For a woman

- are your periods regular?
- what sort of contraceptives have you used in the past?
- have you had a previous pregnancy?
- have you had a miscarriage or termination?

Some doctors will ask you about the number of previous partners you have had, and may also ask questions to establish that you are having sex in the right way. It is a sad fact that every year a few couples still turn up in specialist infertility clinics only for it to be discovered that they have never actually had vaginal intercourse. Your doctor may also want to know if there's anything in your family history that might indicate a problem, such as inherited chromosomal disorders.

Some GPs will take a long time over these questions. Others may feel it is of more benefit to establish the basic facts, then immediately move on to actual testing to establish whether there is a problem or not.

QUESTIONS TO ASK YOUR GP

- do you think we have reason to be concerned?
- what tests do you think should be carried out?
- can you carry out those tests?
- do you think we need to be referred on to a specialist?

If your doctor starts describing where he thinks the problem might lie, or what tests you might need, ask about any terms or suggestions you don't understand. In fact don't be afraid to ask any question of your GP or specialist – there is no such thing as a 'stupid' question when it comes to infertility. Most doctors would rather you asked about anything you are worried or unsure about than have you go away fretting. Amanda worried for ages whether she should ask her GP if she could possibly have had an infection that she didn't know about which might now be affecting her fertility.

'On the face of it, it seems pretty strange, doesn't it? I mean, you usually know when you're ill because you get a temperature, feel sick, go to bed . . . But I'd had my appendix out when I was small and I'd read there was sometimes a chance that infection could get in and I might not even remember this. My GP was able to reassure me that, while it was unlikely, it was something they could look for. I felt much better having got my worry out into the open, and felt more confident that if this was my problem, they'd be alerted into looking for it more closely.'

IF YOUR GP IS UNSUPPORTIVE

Some GPs are better than others in recognising that there may be a serious problem. Caroline realised after a while that her GP was not taking her concerns seriously.

'After a year of trying, and keeping charts, the doctor took a quick glance at them and told me that I was probably ovulating and there

was no cause for concern. He told me to come back in six months if I was still worried. In six months I went back, showed him my charts, and he told me that I was probably ovulating and there was no cause for concern, and to come back in six months. . . . I realised that if I did come back in six months, he would just give me the same answer over again. I pointed out that I was now 33 and didn't feel there was any point in delaying things any longer, and he eventually agreed to give me a blood test to check that I was ovulating. I'm sure that if I hadn't pushed, he would have let me go away in the hopes that our problem would just sort itself out. But that would have just meant an extra six months of unnecessary delay, because later tests showed that I was hardly ovulating at all.'

Jayne's experience also shows that it is not wise to wait too long if you believe there is a problem.

'Our GP told us to wait for two years, which seemed reasonable as I was only 24 at the time. But when we did go back, we found there was an 18-month wait for a hospital appointment, so we had to wait even longer, which was worse because by then we were sure that there was something wrong but we didn't know what it might be or how to deal with it.'

If your GP is really not ready to help when you believe you have a problem, it may be a good idea to contact one of the national support organisations (see p. 278) for advice. If necessary you can change your GP, and they can give advice on this.

POSSIBLE PROBLEM AREAS

As we have seen, conception and pregnancy depend on a range of factors:

- the woman must ovulate
- her fallopian tubes must be open

- the man needs to produce enough live, normal sperm
- these sperm need to get into the vagina and through the cervical mucus
- one sperm must be capable of fertilising the egg
- the resulting embryo must implant successfully
- the woman's hormones and uterus must maintain the pregnancy

As Amanda puts it,

'Once I started reading up about it, I was amazed that anyone ever got pregnant at all – there were so many things that could get in the way. I began to think that waiting for the stork and finding babies under a blackberry bush were much more reliable methods.'

If a couple are not getting pregnant, something may be going wrong at any one of the stages leading up to pregnancy . . .

Ovulation

All sorts of things can interfere with ovulation. If not all the hormones are managing their balancing act precisely, the egg may not mature – or, if it does mature, it may not be released from the follicle (known as luteinised unruptured follicle syndrome). Underactivity of the thyroid gland can also disrupt the endocrine system, leading to ovulation problems.

While many women have polycystic ovaries (polycystic simply means 'many cysts' – small capsules of fluid or fat on the ovaries) this does not necessarily affect fertility. Polycystic ovarian syndrome (PCOS), however, is a condition in which the body is in a state of hormone imbalance, partly because all these cysts are secreting hormones, and this can severely affect fertility.

Fallopian tubes

One of the most common causes of a woman's fertility problems is damage to the fallopian tubes. The damage may have been caused by a past infection (perhaps from having used an IUD), previous surgery in the pelvic area (such as having your appendix out) which has left adhesions and scarring, or by endometriosis. All of these can lead to blockage of the fallopian tubes, or damage to the delicate membranes within the tubes. Tests may show that both your fallopian tubes are completely blocked, so sperm could never reach the egg – but often a fallopian tube is only partially blocked, or one tube is blocked while the other tube is open. These partial blockages reduce fertility and could also trap an egg that does get fertilised, which can lead to an ectopic pregnancy (in which the egg implants not in the uterus but elsewhere, often in the fallopian tubes).

Sometimes a woman will know she has had a past infection which may have caused damage to her tubes; sometimes she won't. An infection from chlamydia, for example, sometimes produces no discernible symptoms, so the fact that it has damaged the tubes may come as a complete surprise. This is why a check on the state of the fallopian tubes is essential in any investigation of infertility.

Similarly, endometriosis is not always easily diagnosed. With this condition, endometrial cells, which usually only line the walls of the uterus, grow elsewhere within the pelvis, often over the ovaries or fallopian tubes. Responding to the hormonal cycle, these cells thicken and then break down each month, but, because the cells are trapped within the pelvic area and cannot be shed, they become sticky and spread. As they spread, they can form swellings or adhesions which join organs to each other, or to the pelvic wall, and can cause blockage of the fallopian tubes. Endometriosis affects an estimated 2 million women in the UK. The causes are still not known and there is no simple cure.

It's a disease that causes varying levels of pain and distress, and the link between the severity of the disease and the pain it causes is not constant. You can have 'mild' endo, yet still suffer devastating pain. Equally, some women are unaware they have the condition until they realise that intercourse never results in a pregnancy, and then tests might show that severe endo has blocked their fallopian tubes. The link with fertility itself is also not clear-cut: many women with endometriosis know they have it because of the pain it causes them, yet they do become pregnant. Others will not. However, if it is not treated, the 'endo' will become a chronic cause of pain and, for many women, infertility.

Sperm

To be in with a good chance of being able to father a child, a man needs to be producing enough sperm, which are able to move forward, and enough of them have to be normal (there are always some that aren't). Although the links between sperm numbers, density, movement and fertility aren't yet fully established, they give a good guide to the chances of a particular man being able to produce enough sperm of good enough quality to fertilise an egg. It's been established that sperm counts are falling in the developed world, so more and more men are facing fertility problems.

As with women, hormone imbalances can severely affect fertility in men. Insufficient levels of hormones can affect sperm production and development, but sometimes a man doesn't produce any sperm at all (this is sometimes referred to as 'idiopathic oligospermia') and the reason why simply can't be found.

There may also be a physical obstruction at various points in the male reproductive system, which is blocking sperm from getting out. The vas deferens may have been damaged during surgery for hernia repair, for example, or the testicles may have been damaged, either through injury, such as from being hit, or as the result of having mumps, or there may be a varicocoele (a swollen vein, which may be visible); varicocoeles don't, however, always affect fertility.

There is also a condition called retrograde ejaculation which can be caused by certain drugs, previous surgery or nerve damage (for example, from diabetes). Sperm simply go in the wrong direction and end up in the bladder rather than the semen. Very rarely, there is an anatomical abnormality which affects fertility. In the condition known as hypospadias, the urethra usually comes out on the underside of the penis. Some men are born without a vas deferens.

In addition, in some cases immunological factors are at work. It seems as if the man's immune system reacts to his sperm as if it were a foreign body like bacteria, and begins to produce antibodies to attack it. The reasons for this are unknown, though immunological factors are currently one of the most intense areas of research in the infertility field.

Cervical mucus

Problems sometimes occur when each partner's system is working well but together they are incompatible. The seminal fluid is alkaline, to counteract the acidic environment of the vagina. Sometimes, however, the chemistry isn't right and the acid secretions of the vagina 'kill off' the sperm on their journey to the egg. This is known, charmingly, as 'hostile' mucus.

Both men and women can have immune reactions to sperm, although little is known about how prevalent a problem this might be for infertile couples. If there are antibodies in either the semen or the cervical mucus, or both, the sperm just can't get through.

Fertilisation

Some sperm appear quite normal under the microscope, using all the usual assessments for normality, motility and so on, but seem to have some chemical, possibly chromosomal, abnormality that means they are not capable of fertilising the egg. As a woman ages, the eggs she produces are also more likely to contain chromosomal or chemical abnormalities, rendering fertilisation impossible. One woman said to me that she had been told her only problem was 'old eggs'.

Implantation

Sometimes the woman's endometrium does not develop thickly enough for an embryo to implant. This can be caused by low progesterone levels, sometimes associated with a condition called luteal phase defect (LPD) in which either the luteal phase of the cycle is too short to allow sufficient progesterone to be produced, or progesterone production is low because the corpus luteum begins to break down too quickly, and the embryo cannot implant properly.

Occasionally a woman may have uterine abnormalities which interfere with successful implantation. There may be problems from DES exposure, septums (bands of tissue dividing the uterus), or a T- or heart-shaped uterus, or no uterus at all. Fibroids can sometimes be present in the uterus, but these do not always affect fertility.

Sustaining the pregnancy

Miscarriage is a devastating event whether it happens early or late in a pregnancy. The reasons for miscarriage vary, and these are looked at in more detail in Chapter 8.

TESTING TIMES

What precisely is going wrong at any of the stages mentioned above is what the tests you may be offered are designed to determine. If the exact reasons why you are not conceiving are investigated thoroughly, you are more likely to get the treatment which is most suitable for you.

Your GP may carry out some of the preliminary tests described below. Most doctors, for example, are able to organise sperm analyses and blood tests to check hormone levels. If at any stage you are referred by your GP to a specialist infertility clinic or gynae-cologist, it is a good idea to ask what tests the clinic or hospital carry out as a routine part of their investigations. If your GP has already arranged for some of these tests to be carried out, ask whether it is necessary to repeat them (especially if you have to pay for them). If you have already undergone some investigations, a specialist clinic may undertake some new ones.

It's a good idea for a couple to be tested at the same time, although many investigations will begin with hormone tests for the woman. However, most doctors and clinics will insist that the man has a semen sample analysed before the woman goes through any invasive physical tests.

The experience of tests for infertility can be very frightening, although Marion found that

'The nights I stayed awake worrying over something that was going to happen the next day were usually much worse than going through it.'

Another thing to keep in mind about infertility investigations is that the process may take a long time. There can be long waiting lists for appointments, which can be difficult to cope with. Sylvia says:

'I felt like we were just wasting time waiting for these dates to come round. They were my only hope and the time seemed to pass so slowly.'

This is why, at some point in the process, many couples decide to dip into the private system where waiting lists for tests and treatments are shorter. Of course, whether you are able to do this depends entirely on your ability to pay.

Basic physical examination

This is the first test you may undergo, possibly by your GP, to check for signs of infection as well as any obvious physical abnormalities. Rarely does a pelvic examination reveal anything untoward, but sometimes it does. Janice was told rather abruptly by her GP that an initial examination revealed that she had 'a deformity' and she would need further tests:

'I felt sick. The word "deformity" made me feel like I was harbouring something ugly and misshapen inside me.'

She later discovered that her cervix was blocked by a large fibroid and she needed surgery to remove the blockage.

It's not exactly pleasant to have someone feeling around inside you and pressing on your stomach, and physical exams aren't always carried out with a great deal of sensitivity to your feelings. Amanda was told, 'Your cervix is very difficult to reach,' as it was quite far back in her vagina. She felt it necessary to inform future doctors of this when they started a physical exam, to try and cut down on their exasperation and her own discomfort.

The GP may check that the man's testicles have descended properly (otherwise the sperm will not be cool enough to develop in sufficient quality and quantity), check for varicocoeles and examine the prostate gland for signs of infection.

Semen analysis

For this test, a man will be given a sterile container and a set of forms to fill in, giving details of the date and time the sample was produced. He will have to masturbate directly into the container, and, if he's done the test at home, deliver it to the laboratory himself within the hour, keeping it warm on the way.

A 'good' test will show that:

- the volume (amount) of seminal fluid is greater than 2ml
- sperm density is more than 20 million per ml
- more than 40 per cent of the sperm have normal motility and are moving forward

- at least 70 per cent of the sperm have normal morphology (are not abnormally shaped)[2]

If there's any 'clumping together', further tests may be carried out to check for antisperm antibodies. The main factor is whether enough normal sperm have good motility – this seems to be more important than the numbers themselves. Once your doctors have the results of the analysis another test will probably be carried out, especially if the results were poor, since sperm count varies.

Finding out that your sperm doesn't achieve the desired standards can come as a great shock. After all, most semen looks pretty similar and it's impossible to judge it by appearance. To find out that it contains no sperm at all, for example, can be a devastating discovery and it can take a couple a long time to recover from such news.

Quite often people are too upset by the results of a semen analysis to ask all the questions they want to, or questions may only occur to them later. If you don't feel you had enough time to absorb the implications of the analysis, go back and see your doctor again to talk it through. There are ways forward, though it may not seem like it at the time.

The analysis may be followed by two additional tests. In the 'swim-up' test, the sperm are put in a tube and covered by a special fluid. Only normal sperm will swim up into the fluid. This test allows the percentage of normal sperm to be established (and is also sometimes used as part of artificial insemination treatment to separate out the strongest swimmers). The velocity of sperm is sometimes also measured separately, using microscopic photography to check the distance the sperm travel.

Hormone levels

These are simple blood tests to check if there is a hormonal imbalance. For a woman, they are usually carried out around Day 21 of your cycle when they can indicate whether you have ovulated. The levels of most of the hormones known to play a part in fertility are checked, including testosterone, oestrogen, progesterone, FSH (follicle-stimulating hormone), LH (luteinising hormone), prolactin and the thyroid hormone thyroxine.

The levels of various hormones for a woman can indicate where a problem might lie: elevated LH levels may indicate polycystic ovary syndrome; high FSH may indicate premature ovarian failure. High levels of prolactin (which stimulates the production of breastmilk) may lead to irregular ovulation. Low levels of progesterone may indicate that an embryo is unlikely to implant because the endometrium isn't thick enough. Everyone's hormone test levels will be different, and before moving on you need to discuss carefully with your doctor what each hormone level means not only on its own but also in combination.

Some patterns of hormone abnormalities are more amenable to treatment than others. For example, lowering prolactin levels can be achieved with Bromocriptine. Others will need a more complicated and sometimes more aggressive therapy.

Hormone abnormalities affecting sperm production include thyroid problems, low testosterone levels, elevated FSH and excess prolactin.

Post-coital test

This test checks the cervical mucus for presence of sperm after intercourse. Using a speculum, a sample of cervical fluid is obtained from the cervix a few hours after intercourse. This must take place around the time of ovulation, when a woman has 'fertile' mucus; otherwise the test results won't be worth much because ordinary 'non-fertile' mucus is highly resistant to sperm. The mucus is then checked under a microscope to see if motile sperm are present. If a high number are dead, there's obviously a problem. It's obviously a very useful test, because it shows what is happening inside the body after sex and can indicate if a 'hostile' reaction is taking place.

This test sounds very simple in theory but, as soon as you start to think about it, you realise how horrendously complicated it is in practice. First you have to have sex on medical demand – about eight hours before you're booked in to go to the hospital – and you've also got to assess whether you are in fact within your 'fertile' days when the appointment comes around. If you're sure you're not ovulating, you can ring up and change the appointment, but quite often you simply won't be certain.

Leona says:

'Our doctor told us he wanted to do a post-coital test, and we'd need to have sex around the time of ovulation and so on and so on, and I just looked at him in amazement. I never know when I'm ovulating, so how were we supposed to time this correctly?'

Leona's cervical mucus changes were minimal, her cycle was irregular, and she had found that OPKs did not always give her clear readings. This is not an uncommon problem, and if a test is done when the mucus is thick and not letting much sperm through the results can make a couple feel disconsolate when they don't need to be. If this is the case for you, suggest the test is repeated another month, when signals are clearer.

Sperm invasion test

If the post-coital test shows that the sperm aren't getting through, it may be followed by the sperm invasion test. A sample of your cervical mucus (again, taken at around the time of ovulation) is placed on a laboratory slide with a drop of your partner's semen next to it. Another slide is placed on top, which brings the two liquids into contact. Examination under a microscope can then show how far the sperm are penetrating into the mucus. If, for example, the sperm are normal but clump together and don't move forward in the cervical mucus, or if they look normal but are dead by the time they have moved through the mucus, there is obviously something going wrong and it may be because one of you is producing antibodies. These can be either autoimmune (the man is producing antibodies to his own sperm) or alloimmune (the woman is producing them). If this is the case, a 'crossover' test may be done, in which the man's semen is put on a slide with someone else's mucus and your mucus is put on a slide with someone else's semen. This can show whether the problem lies with just one of you, or whether there is only a problem when your particular fluids come in contact.

Your mucus may also be analysed to see if it 'ferns' under a microscope. This is a check to ensure that your hormones are working to make it as stretchy as it needs to be to let sperm through.

Testing for infection or disorder

Some doctors recommend that you have a test for a variety of infections including gonorrhoea, chlamydia, syphilis, toxoplasmosis, rubella, cytomegalovirus, hepatitis B and C, and HIV. A urinalysis may look for signs of a urinary tract infection, the presence of sperm in the urine (which, with a low sperm count, may indicate retrograde ejaculation), and signs of systemic disorders such as kidney problems or diabetes.

Physical investigations

Most investigative and invasive physical tests on a woman, such as laparoscopy and HSG, are usually scheduled for early in the cycle in order to avoid interrupting any unsuspected developing pregnancy (although a laparoscopy designed to deal with endometriosis may well be scheduled for post-ovulation days, when the extent of the condition may be easier to ascertain). If yours isn't, you may want to try to get the date changed. Being realistic, though, you may not get much choice about surgery schedules.

Laparoscopy

In this procedure, carried out under general anaesthetic, a small incision is made in the woman's abdomen, usually just under the navel, through which a laparoscope (an illuminated viewing tube with a tiny camera at one end) can be inserted. The abdomen is inflated with carbon dioxide to make the uterus, ovaries and tubes easier to see. A laparoscopy allows a surgeon to look for structural abnormalities, endometriosis and adhesions, and possibly to put right any problems at the same time. The operation is also carried out in many hospitals as a standard way of assessing whether the fallopian tubes are open: if dye is injected through the cervix, it should be seen flowing out of the ends of the tubes. If it doesn't, they're blocked. It's usually carried out as a day procedure, although some hospitals prefer to keep you in overnight.

While it is only a minor surgical procedure, any operation throws some women into blind panic. Carmel, booked in for a laparoscopy next month, says:

'I am very nervous about the lap. In fact, it's the anaesthetic more than the surgery that bothers me. I've never had an anaesthetic before.'

Liz, too, thought she was coping very well with her infertility until she was told she'd need a laparoscopy to check for endometriosis 'and nearly fainted'.

Diane found the night before she was due to go in for her laparoscopy very worrying. Her consultant had suggested the test because he thought she might have polycystic ovary syndrome, and wanted to check that nothing else was amiss:

'For me, this was terrifying. I had never been in hospital before, and now I was faced with going in for an operation that might tell me that I might never have children. When I was told that the lap had given me the all-clear, the relief was overwhelming.'

A laparoscopy carries the small risks and potential side-effects of any procedure which requires a general anaesthetic, and you may find it takes a while to recover. You may feel some soreness in your abdomen for a few days afterwards, and sometimes intense pain from the carbon dioxide that's been blown into your abdomen and is now trying to 'escape', and sometimes you may have some vaginal bleeding and also heavy vaginal secretions as the dye leaks out. As if that wasn't enough, you may also have a sore throat because of the tube inserted by the anaesthetist. If you are worried about any symptoms you may experience, always contact the hospital or clinic where the operation was carried out.

Despite its drawbacks, a lap can provide a great deal of useful information about your body, and the tiny scar will fade almost to invisibility.

Hysterosalpingography (HSG)

The main purpose of this test is to check whether the fallopian tubes are open. A catheter is inserted through the woman's cervix and a small amount of dye is injected through it into the uterus. If there are no blockages, the dye will move into the fallopian tubes as well. This dye shows up on X-rays and so allows the shape of the uterus to be observed, and the way the dye flows through the fallopian tubes will show if there are any blockages there. To avoid the risks of radiation to an unsuspected pregnancy, an HSG should only be carried out in the first ten days of the cycle. The test is usually done in the hospital's X-ray department and you can go home soon afterwards.

This is a very useful and worthwhile test as it can show im-mediately if there's a problem, but it can cause mild to severe cramps like period pains. Be ready for that, and if you are tense take a painkiller in advance. Alice found her test 'very interesting' if nerve-racking, and she has had the procedure done twice.

'It only took a few minutes each time. The doctor injected the dye through my cervix and I could see on a screen where it was going. It

didn't hurt at all, though the second time I did get some uncomfortable feelings when they were opening up my cervix, but it didn't last long.'

Sylvia found her test more painful:

'They said I might feel some cramps, like period pains, but opening up the cervix caused more pain than I was prepared for. If some women really do have period pains like that, then I sympathise with them wholeheartedly. But the nurses were wonderful and very supportive and helped me get through.'

However, more than one woman, when I spoke to them about this test, immediately came up with the word 'excruciating'. How much discomfort you will experience will undoubtedly depend on who's doing the test, how it's done and how tense you are, but it cannot be denied that some women feel a great deal of pain from an HSG. Gail says:

'I wish someone had told me of the pain I might experience so I would know it wasn't just me. You need to be prepared for these things. It may not hurt. But I also know that some doctors prefer to carry this test out under general anaesthesia because of the pain it can cause.'

If it hurts, let the hospital staff know. It may simply be because they're not being as gentle as they should be.

Take someone with you for support if you can, as this can reduce your stress levels and make the procedure less uncomfortable, although they won't be allowed in the room with you because of the risks from the radiation. Also, you probably won't feel like driving yourself home afterwards, so arrange for another driver or alternative means of transport.

One of the main advantages of an HSG over a laparoscopy is that you avoid the need for a general anaesthetic and surgery. There are also potential hidden benefits with an HSG. Julie says:

*'I knew they increased your chances of conceiving because they sort of
clear out the tubes. So I kept my fingers crossed, and about three months
after the dye test I did get pregnant.'*

Hysteroscopy

The cervix is dilated just enough to insert a small scope which
allows the doctor to look at the inside of the uterus. Minor
abnormalities such as polyps or adhesions can be treated during
this procedure, which can be done under local or general anaesthesia. It may also show the presence of fibroids, but as these don't
necessarily interfere with fertility, your doctor may advise you that
there is no need to remove them surgically. You may have some
vaginal bleeding afterwards, but few women report any lasting
pain.

Hysterosalpingo-contrast sonography (HyCoSy)

This is a relatively new test for assessing whether the fallopian tubes
are open. A contrast medium (a sugar solution) is injected through
the cervix in conjunction with transvaginal ultrasound scanning.
The contrast solution outlines the shape of the uterus, allowing any
abnormalities to be seen, and the flow of the solution along the
tubes can be traced. It can also show up any cysts or endometriosis
on the ovaries. The procedure takes between 15 and 30 minutes
and you can go home straight afterwards. If it does show up
potential problems you may need a further laparoscopy, but this
can be planned to deal with the problem (rather than, as often
happens, having an initial laparoscopy which shows up a problem
and then coming back later for further surgery to deal with the
problem). However, it is not appropriate for everyone and your
doctor may recommend a laparoscopy for a full assessment of your
pelvic cavity. Nevertheless, if it is appropriate, it avoids the risks
and worry associated with general anaesthesia. As with the other
tests, you may feel some period-like cramps and discomfort, so you
may like to take a painkiller in advance.

Ultrasound scanning

Abdominal ultrasound, in which a transducer is passed over the skin of the abdomen, can give a picture of the uterus and ovaries. Fibroids and uterine abnormalities may be visible, and polycystic ovary syndrome can be diagnosed if ultrasound shows many cysts in the ovaries. Ultrasound can also monitor the development of eggs in the ovaries and can show the failure of a follicle to release an egg even though it has reached maturity. This can be a very interesting test, not least because you get to see the images on the screen, although you may not be able to make much sense of them. Amanda thought her reproductive equipment looked like 'a cold weather front'. One uncomfortable aspect of the test, if it's being done abdominally, is that you have to have a full bladder to enable the ovaries to be seen clearly. This may mean you're concentrating so much on not wetting yourself that you can't concentrate on the images on the screen anyway.

Gail found it a very uncomfortable procedure:

'They were poking and prodding me about. The nurse said to me, "Well, we can't find your ovaries," as if it was my fault that they had gone missing in the night.'

Sometimes transvaginal ultrasound, in which a transducer wand is inserted through the vagina, is used to view the cervix, uterus and ovaries because it can provide greater detail than abdominal ultrasound. Gilli remembers:

'As I watched the doctor put a condom over this thing ready to put it into my vagina, I thought it would be funny if I didn't have to experience it myself.'

One advantage is you don't have to have a full bladder for this method of scanning.

For a man, ultrasound of the seminal vesicles can show their size, development, and whether they are storing and passing on sperm properly.

Endometrial biopsy
A small catheter is inserted through the cervix and a small sample (biopsy) of the uterine lining is removed. This is done two or three days before your period is due. The sample can then be analysed to check whether your endometrium has thickened, as would be expected, in preparation for the implantation of an embryo. If it has not developed as expected for that phase of your cycle, this can indicate a problem with progesterone levels. The test can also be used to check for infection, too, although if this is suspected a D&C (dilatation and curettage – a scraping of the endometrium under general anaesthetic) may be needed.

Surgical exploration of the testes
This is a test of last resort and only carried out if no other reason can be found for a man's infertility. Exploration can check for blockages or infections, and a biopsy may be taken: the doctor takes a small piece of testicular tissue and checks the sperm-producing tubules and the cells between them. If the tubules and the sperm in them are normal (but a semen analysis showed no sperm), the problem is likely to be a blockage elsewhere. A vasogram may be performed if a blockage is suspected; dye is injected into the vas deferens and under X-rays this will outline the ducts and pinpoint any obstructions. A biopsy may also show that the sperm are not maturing properly or that no sperm are being produced.

Other tests

In addition to the basic tests, there are many others that are not always used, as many health professionals feel they are of doubtful diagnostic value or unproven worth in particular cases. The hamster egg test, for example, assesses the ability of a man's sperm to penetrate a specially prepared hamster egg. This test is of controversial benefit, as there is no clear evidence that the results indicate whether the sperm can also fertilise a human egg.

What you are offered will depend on what your consultant feels is most appropriate for your own circumstances.

At any point in the testing programme, ask whatever questions you need. Too often, people will assume you know things when you don't. Gail found this very frustrating:

'Things were never explained. It was always like I didn't matter.'

WHAT NEXT?

When you've been through one, two, some or all of the tests to try to discover why you are not conceiving, you will be told:

- there is **definitely something wrong** (such as a man producing no sperm), which means that you won't be able to get pregnant without further treatment, however long you wait, or however often you have sex; or
- there is something that is having **a mild effect** on your fertility (like irregular ovulation or endometriosis) but it's possible you could still get pregnant without intervention, although it may take a little longer; or
- **they don't know** why you're not conceiving. Again, you could still conceive, but you may not

Perhaps being told a definite reason why you are not conceiving is easier. You can then find out about the treatments on offer which will try to cure, solve or get round the problem, and then decide whether you want to go ahead with these. If there is something which is having a mild effect on your fertility, the process of weighing up the costs and benefits of possible treatments is more difficult, but at least you know what you're dealing with.

Despite the battery of tests now available, one of the most

common forms of infertility – for as many as 30 per cent of couples, according to the Human Fertilisation and Embryology Authority (HFEA) – is 'unexplained' infertility: when there is no apparent physical or hormonal cause for a couple's not conceiving. As Karen says,

'It's always easier to cope if you understand what's going on, if you know what the reason is. If they can't give you a reason, you're left in the wilderness without a map.'

If you have 'unexplained' infertility, it doesn't mean there isn't a reason why you're not conceiving – just that doctors haven't been able to identify it yet. In addition, it can often be treated successfully through techniques such as IVF, which may bypass whatever the hidden problem was. However, when the reason you are not conceiving is not clear, it can be much more difficult to decide what to do next.

It can also be difficult to decide because we can't always take in the information all at once, or come up with all the right questions immediately when our test results come through, even if the doctor does sit down and explain everything carefully. Diane says,

'I made so many notes about our test results, and wrote down all the things we'd have to think about very neatly in a notebook I'd brought with me, and I nodded and smiled, and it was only when I got home I realised I'd hardly taken in a word of it because I was just so shocked that we might really have a serious problem. I looked at all my neat writing and broke down in tears.'

There are very many things to take into consideration when deciding what to do next. You will want to consider:

- whether you want to go ahead with treatment at all
- what treatments you could receive on the NHS
- what treatments you could access as a private patient
- what the impact of treatment on you as a couple might be

All these factors are considered in Chapter 4.

Before going ahead with a particular treatment, you will also want to know much more about what the treatment itself involves. This is looked at in detail in Chapter 5.

4

Where Do We Go from Here?

Different causes of infertility require different approaches. If you understand fully the reasons for your infertility, where they can be identified, you will have a greater understanding of why a particular treatment is being offered to you and how likely it is to be able to help you. Below is an overview of some of the treatments you may be offered, to give you an idea of what may be suggested for you and help put your decision-making in context. Each of the treatments is covered in more detail in Chapter 5.

FEMALE FACTOR INFERTILITY

- if the woman has irregular or infrequent ovulation, stimulatory drugs such as clomiphene may resolve this problem
- if she has luteal phase problems (for example, not enough progesterone), drug support after ovulation may be of benefit
- if she doesn't ovulate at all, donor eggs may be needed for in vitro fertilisation (IVF) treatment
- if her fallopian tubes are blocked they may be repaired through tubal microsurgery, or IVF may be needed if they are seriously damaged
- if she has endometriosis, surgery or laser treatment could be used to clear it, or drug therapy may be appropriate
- if she has a chromosomal disorder, she may need to consider IVF using donor eggs, or surrogacy

- if she has uterine problems or no uterus, the couple will need to consider surrogacy using the woman's own or donated eggs

MALE FACTOR INFERTILITY

- a physical obstruction preventing the sperm from reaching the semen may be corrected through microsurgery, or sperm may be extracted through a surgical procedure and used in IVF
- if the man isn't producing any sperm, or the sperm he does produce aren't fertile, the couple will need to consider assisted conception using donor sperm
- if he has a low sperm count, the couple could consider assisted conception using his own sperm (in techniques such as artificial insemination (AI) or intrauterine insemination) (IUI). If the sperm count is very low, ICSI (intracytoplasmic sperm injection) may be a suitable treatment
- if he has a chromosomal disorder, the couple may need to consider AI or IVF using donor sperm
- if a man is producing antibodies to his own sperm, this may be overcome with IUI once his sperm has been treated

JOINT INFERTILITY

- in some cases, a couple's inability to conceive is caused by problems with the sperm getting through the cervical mucus, which could be overcome with AI/IUI using the man's sperm
- difficulties with intercourse may also mean that AI is a good way forward
- if a woman is producing antibodies to her partner's sperm, IUI may be enough to overcome the problem, although IVF may be required

UNEXPLAINED INFERTILITY

- if the couple's infertility is unexplained (i.e. the doctors just can't work out why you're not conceiving) GIFT or IVF may be of benefit, possibly using donor sperm or eggs

This isn't an exhaustive list of either conditions or treatment options. You will always need to discuss with your doctor what is best for you and your particular circumstances. Many couples will find that they have a combination of problems, such as irregular ovulation plus a low sperm count, or infrequent ovulation plus problems with the thickening of the endometrium. In addition, new techniques in assisted conception are constantly being developed and your doctor may feel that one of these is appropriate for you. When deciding whether to go forward or not, however, the first thing you will need to do is come to terms with the nature of your problem.

COMING TO TERMS WITH YOUR DIAGNOSIS

When a particular problem is diagnosed you may find this actually helpful, as Maria did:

'We now knew what we were dealing with, and knew that there were particular treatments for polycystic ovaries. It was much better than being in the dark.'

More often you will have very mixed feelings. Gilli says,

'When tests showed that the problem lay with me I felt a sense of relief because I knew that female problems, especially hormone problems, were easier to treat. But at the same time what a terrible sense of failure: my body wasn't working properly and I was letting my partner down in such a fundamental way.'

If you're diagnosed with endometriosis, as many women under-going investigations will be, you will need to consider carefully what to do. Sometimes drug therapy is recommended, which puts a temporary stop to the production of some of your fertility hormones for several months in the hope that the endo will dissolve. Sometimes the endo can be removed by laser, which will increase your chances of getting pregnant. In severe cases, your doctor may even recommend surgery on your uterus or ovaries.

What you decide to do will depend on your age, how long you've been trying to conceive, and how badly the endo affects your life. There's no 'right' answer. What you can do is make sure that you're seen by an endo specialist who understands both the disease and fertility issues, and ask for a second opinion if you're unsure about the course you're advised to take. Contact the Endometriosis Society (see p.279) for more advice if you need to.

Tanya, who was found to have severe endo blocking both her tubes, was extremely dismayed by the diagnosis.

'I felt like a woman whose body wasn't working properly, like a second-class citizen, like I was defective.'

She got a lot of support from the Endometriosis Society's helpline;

'I talked to someone who made me feel that it wasn't me being defective, just a problem we would now know how to deal with'

but even so found her sense of despondency hard to shake off.

Similarly, Sylvia, whose tubes were found to be damaged and who was told she would need help to conceive, admits to being 'taken aback' by the discovery.

'It feels like my life has suddenly gone out of my control. We never thought it would really come to this. I'm finding it very difficult to accept that the only way we'll ever have children is through technology.'

Accepting the fact that you will definitely need treatment may take some time, as Kate and Mike found when they discovered that Mike was not producing any sperm.

'We were devastated by Mike's infertility. We'd begun our marriage blithely anticipating becoming parents. Like most of our generation, we believed our fertility was within our control and it was a shock to find it wasn't. After the results of the test came through, we needed time to mourn for the family we would never create together.'

Of course, if you've been through every test available and still no one knows why you're not conceiving, it can be particularly hard to take, as Caroline found:

'It wasn't just for ourselves, although it would have been so much better if we could have been given a clear explanation, but it would have helped us to deal with other people around us, too. They knew we'd gone for all these tests and couldn't believe they hadn't turned up any cause. I definitely got the feeling they thought we weren't getting pregnant because we were thinking about it too much.'

Rachel, whose fertility is also 'unexplained', remembers that there was a joke going round her patient support group, although they would never have let the medical staff in on it.

'It goes something like "How many fertility experts does it take to have a clue?" If you can't keep your sense of humour, you're done for.'

SHOULD YOU HAVE TREATMENT?

It's important to take time out as a couple once you know the results of the initial tests. Just because infertility treatments may be available, it doesn't mean that you have to make use of them. Powerful medical techniques carry risk as well as hope. Whether you decide to avail yourself of what may be offered must ultimately be your decision.

Anne feels that

'Although I'm very glad that the technology does exist, I'm very disappointed that we're going to have to make use of it.'

Carol, too has doubts.

'These are all such relatively new treatments that I know nobody can predict all the long-term effects. You read some very scary stories. I've got so many uncertainties and I'm not sure all my questions could be answered unless I waited round for a hundred years. Not a very plausible solution when I'm already 34 and time is of the essence.'

You will need to consider both the emotional and financial implications of moving forward. Your GP can put you in touch with a counsellor if you want to talk things through, and you will definitely be offered counselling if you've been referred for IVF or treatment involving donor gametes. However, Carol suggests that you sit down with your partner once you know what your problem might be – even if it's 'unexplained' – and work out what you would both want to do before moving on to the next stage.

'It's very important to work out your limits, both financially and emotionally, and you can't always assume that they will be the same for both of you. It's no good getting yourself referred to a clinic for ICSI if you know you won't be able to afford it. And it's no good looking into DI if either one of you has a problem with that. It's best to know these things before you begin, otherwise you might find yourself going along with people's suggestions and then falling apart because you're un-happy.'

Unfortunately, even if you're both happy about moving on to the treatment considered best for you, issues such as waiting lists or your ability to pay will often influence what you do next.

Hold on to your hopes

Everyone has the right to be assessed for infertility treatment. But not all couples will be deemed by their health authority eligible for treatment, and some health authorities offer no help at all to infertile couples.

WHAT CAN THE NHS OFFER ME?

At the moment, with no central guidance on what health authorities should offer, the availability of treatment on the NHS is a lottery. What will be available depends on where you live, which is why many couples with fertility problems talk of the 'babies by postcode' rule that seems to apply. Many health authorities make no funding available for infertility treatment. In other places, what is available will be strictly rationed. For example:

- drug treatment may be available but nothing else
- you may be able to have fertility treatment such as GIFT, but not IVF
- you may be able to have tubal microsurgery but not IVF
- some health authorities will fund a maximum of three cycles of IVF

This means that even if your health authority does fund infertility treatment, it may not fund the treatment your doctor has recommended for you. Most health authorities that do fund will offer ovulation induction treatments and tubal surgery, but they may not offer IVF. This means that you could end up being offered a treatment which is not the right one for you.

In addition, each health authority has its own criteria which determine *who* they will fund for which treatment. You may find, for example, if you need IVF treatment, that you will need to be:

- married with no children
- within a certain age bracket (which will vary)

Criteria for other treatments, even within the same health authority, may be different. Your Community Health Council will have a list of the criteria for treatment in your area. You may also find that some health authorities impose a minimum period of residence within their boundaries before they will fund your treatment; otherwise they might find themselves with an influx of infertile couples moving in from less helpful health authorities. It can be very frustrating to be told you don't qualify for help with funding, especially when you know that if you lived somewhere else you would.

Gail, who is 33, is also uneasy for another reason:

'Our health authority will only fund women aged 35 as they're trying to clear the backlog. I'm worried that by the time I get to 35, they'll have moved the goalposts and I'll be told that I'm too old.'

In particular, many disabled parents need treatment for infertility but may find themselves facing barriers that other couples do not have to confront. Tracy and Robin, who both have disabilities, were pleased when their GP referred them to the local infertility clinic where they met with a wholly positive attitude from the team. Nothing was found to be amiss, so they were referred to a specialist clinic for intrauterine insemination (IUI). There they found a different attitude, Robin remembers:

'We were told that there would probably be quite a wait for treatment and that we would have to be interviewed by the clinic's consultant to ascertain our suitability for treatment. At this point the alarm bells

started ringing as the last thing we needed was some doctor passing moral judgement about our future parenting abilities. As disabled people, we are used to others projecting their moral misrepresentations of our lives and we were warned by friends in a similar situation that we could face some very stiff opposition. After all, who asks the able-bodied population about the quality of life that they, as parents, would provide? Yet, should you have a disabled child, who better than disabled parents to act as positive role models and understand the considerable oppression that they will face? However, after a frank discussion with the consultant, he agreed to put us on the waiting list. Appreciating the progressive nature of Tracy's condition (she has muscular dystrophy), we were enrolled on to the programme some six weeks later.'

WHY IS THE SYSTEM SUCH A LOTTERY?

The inconsistency between health authorities stems partly from the fact that the new technologies for infertility treatment have developed very rapidly and very recently. Once, there was very little help that the medical profession could offer an infertile couple. As techniques like IVF not only became more established but more successful, demand for them began to grow.

Realistically, there will always be rationing of medical treatments. New developments such as ICSI offer great hope to infertile couples, but they are also very expensive. It is therefore inevitable that some health authorities will refuse to help couples for whom this treatment could be very effective, simply because they cannot afford to do so.

Health authorities do come under pressure, as well, from people who feel that no help should ever be given to infertile couples. After all, childlessness is not a life- threatening condition in the way that cancer is. The case for more equitable provision is not helped, either, when stories of people who are judged patently unsuitable for treatment (depending on your point of view, this could range from lesbians to women over 40 to couples where one partner has

HIV to people who already have one child) are paraded in the press.

There will always be cases where it can be difficult to justify spending money on a treatment that is unlikely to work, and there will always be difficult decisions, too. What about a couple who conceive on their third attempt at IUI and then miscarry? They may not be eligible for any more NHS treatment, having received their quota, but the procedure has been proved to work for them once, so they stand a very good chance of conceiving again. As Amanda says,

'We need more rational rationing.'

FINDING A WAY THROUGH THE SYSTEM

In practice, many women shuttle back and forth between NHS and private treatment, as Sophie did:

'My GP thought the local hospital might treat me but there was a long waiting list, and in the meantime I went to see another doctor privately because I wanted to get on with some investigations, and then my appointment came up at the local hospital so I went there for treatment.'

How you weave your way through the system will very much depend what is on offer in your area. Your GP may only be able to refer you to the local gynaecological hospital. They may be able to do some investigations, then refer you somewhere else for treatment or do some treatment themselves and only move you on if you need IVF, for example. Sometimes you can be referred to an infertility specialist straightaway.

You need to be confident that the treatment you are offered by your health authority or by a clinic is appropriate for dealing with the type of infertility you have, and consider whether you want to put yourself through it if there is only a small chance that it will actually help you. Sally and her partner, Daniel, decided to pay for a private medical exam and consultant interview and feel it was worth it.

'Our GP had said he would put us forward for GIFT, which was all our health authority would fund, but we didn't feel it was what we needed. The consultant advised us not to go ahead with the treatment and we feel we saved ourselves a lot of heartache because of this.'

Sometimes you may be lucky enough to be offered treatment, either at no charge or at a reduced cost, if your needs coincide with those of a particular research study. Gail, for example, was offered three attempts at IUI as part of a research programme using a Doppler scanner to measure blood flow to the ovaries.

Alison feels that she and Peter, disabled as the result of a road accident, were incredibly lucky.

'We were put in touch with Bourn Hall just when they were getting involved in a study into spinal cord injuries and the effect that different-level breaks had on fertility. The woman was supposed to be between 20 and 30 and have no problems, so I think we only just got in because I was 31. When we were accepted for the study, we were overjoyed because it meant that fertility treatment wasn't going to cost us anything.'

However, even if your health authority considers you eligible for treatment, there are financial implications, including:

- the hidden costs of taking time off work
- travel costs (you may need to make a lot of journeys to the clinic)
- the costs of any childminding or babysitting if you already have a child

Even if your health authority offers you treatment, you may find that you need to make a financial contribution and this can be substantial. Robin and Tracy didn't have to pay the full cost for their AI treatment, 'just a contribution of £100 a time', but even this was a significant amount for them.

After the initial excitement, more and more health authorities seem to be cutting back on provision for infertile couples, perhaps because demand threatened to increase costs for treatments which have a relatively low success rate (in health budget managers' eyes), although the success rate of one cycle of IVF gives a couple about the same chance of conceiving as having intercourse during one cycle. Gilli echoes the feelings of many when she says,

'I'm so very grateful for the chance of help we were offered. I'm in no doubt that treatment should be given a higher profile in the NHS. No one should be denied the chance of a family because of the cost.'

If you're having difficulty obtaining treatment, you may like to contact the National Infertility Awareness Campaign (see p. 280), which is campaigning for more equitable provision of treatment.

WAITING LISTS

Waiting several months for an appointment or a test is common. By the time you've jumped through all the hoops and they've found a cause for your infertility (or not), several years may have passed – and even one year is critical when you're desperately trying to have a baby. Even after a cause has been diagnosed you may have to wait for treatment to begin.

Mira was eventually diagnosed with severely blocked fallopian tubes.

'The consultant said they couldn't be cleared and suggested we try IVF. This was available on the NHS where we lived, and we would be allowed three attempts, but we had to wait for about a year before treatment could begin. It seemed like such a long time away and I was

worried that our health authority would decide to stop funding the treatment before we got to the top of the list.'

Waiting can be very frustrating. Gilli found that

'Motherhood tantalised me. Babies suddenly seemed to be everywhere, as if there had been a population explosion, but of course it was just that I was acutely aware of parents and their babies now.'

One of the main advantages of private treatment is that, if you have the ability to pay, you can bypass NHS waiting lists altogether, although private clinics sometimes have their own, if shorter, waiting times.

CAN YOU AFFORD PRIVATE TREATMENT?

Amanda says,

'We sent away for information from several treatment centres, and they all came back with glossy brochures and the message that we wouldn't have to wait forever for treatment but could start with our first consultation in a couple of weeks. On the one hand, it was like a dream come true: here were people who could help us and they were only a phone call away. On the other hand, when I looked through the rate cards and saw things like "IUI without scans" and a list of prices, it was the closest I think I've ever felt to thinking we were buying a baby.'

Her partner, Peter, disagrees.

'We weren't buying a baby. I think that was the key. We were buying the chance of having a baby. I'd look at these prices, a couple of thousand pounds, and think that if we could be guaranteed a baby at the end of all this, then we would pay an awful lot more.'

Most clinics offer private treatment to those unable to receive funding through their local health authority, provided they conform to the clinic's own eligibility criteria (there is more about these criteria on page 96). The costs at each clinic will vary: expect to find a difference of several thousand pounds for the same treatment between some clinics.

If your GP is sympathetic and will agree to fund the costs of the drugs you will need for your treatment, this can mean the difference between being able to go ahead with treatment or not. It is worth asking if your GP will do this, as many will.

If you have a private health scheme, enquire whether your insurance will fund any part of the investigations or treatment.

Very many couples, however, are entirely on their own. If you decide that you can afford private treatment, the cost is just one factor to consider. The next is, which clinic should you go to?

CHOOSING A CLINIC

All clinics in the UK which offer IVF or any treatment involving donated sperm or eggs must be licensed by the HFEA, and must keep to the Authority's standards. Nevertheless, the type and range of services offered differ widely, as do their success rates. Clinics offering other treatments, such as IUI or GIFT, don't need to be licensed by the HFEA, but the guidelines below may be useful when choosing which clinic is right for you

All HFEA-licensed clinics must supply written information to couples seeking treatment. This information should give details about:

- the services the clinic offers
- any risks involved
- the costs of treatment
- previous live birth rates
- the clinic's complaints procedure

The leaflets and brochures are usually detailed and fairly easy to read, but always ask if anything seems unclear.

Different clinics will suit different couples; there is no 'best' clinic because so many factors will affect whether a clinic is right for you. You can approach several and make a comparison of what they can offer you, but you also need to take into account some very practical considerations. These considerations also apply if you are receiving NHS funding and have little choice about where you are treated:

- how long will you have to wait for your first consultation appointment with the clinic?
- what treatments can the clinic offer? Some clinics offer a wide variety, which can be an advantage because if one type isn't successful you could try another at the same clinic. Some specialise in one treatment, or in treating one type of infertility, which can be an advantage if that is just what you need
- how long are the waiting lists for the treatment you will need? (For some treatments the waiting times may be much longer than for others; for example, donated eggs are generally in short supply so you might find yourself waiting a very long time if this is what you need.)
- does the clinic have any treatment criteria, such as age limits, which would exclude you?
- how close is the clinic? Treatment can involve a great deal of travelling over a long period of time; this is an important factor, especially if you will have to take time off work for treatment. A clinic that is too far away will add to the stress of your treatment

There are also wider considerations which you may wish to take into account, depending on their importance to you. For example, you may want to have answers to the following questions:

- can you see a woman doctor?
- will you be seen by the same doctor throughout your care?
- what support can the clinic offer? Some have patient support groups which offer a great deal of information while you are considering or undergoing treatment. They can also give you a chance to talk to other people who are having treatment at the same clinic, and provide emotional and psychological support. If there is no patient support group at the clinic you choose, you may like to contact one of the national support groups (see p. 278).
- are any of the clinic's facilities shared with other services, like the maternity unit? This may be good news if your treatment results in a pregnancy, as you can continue to visit the same centre for antenatal care, but may become distressing if you don't conceive and have to sit in a waiting room filled with obviously pregnant women

SUCCESS RATES

The success rate of a clinic will be one of the first things you want to know. The clinic should give you figures relating to the various types of treatment on offer there. You may like to compare these with the national average success rates for treatments of that kind. (The HFEA will be able to provide you with the most recent figures for IVF and DI treatments.)

The outcomes of infertility treatments can be expressed in a variety of ways. The two most commonly used are:

- the live birth rate
- the clinical pregnancy rate

The clinic may tell you these rates for:

- each treatment cycle
- each egg collected

- each embryo transfer
- each patient

However, the HFEA recommends that IVF clinics should tell prospective patients the live birth rate per treatment cycle, often called the 'take-home baby rate'. This figure represents the probability you have of eventually taking home a baby after a single treatment cycle.

Over the past two decades, more and more couples have been making use of IVF and the success rate continues to rise. HFEA data for 1985 shows that in that year 4308 treatment cycles were begun, with a live birth rate per treatment cycle of 8.6 per cent. In the period from 31 January 1995 to 31 March 1996, a total of 36,994 treatment cycles were started (in 26,967 women), and of these treatment cycles 30,354 reached embryo transfer stage. There were 6827 clinical pregnancies and 5542 'live birth events'. The national average success rate was therefore 15 per cent for all treatments started, but individual clinics may achieve higher or lower levels than this.[3]

But don't judge a clinic by its statistics alone. There may be valid reasons why the success rate of one clinic is lower than that of another. The clinic may, for instance, specialise in treating older women, and for women aged 35 and over the chances of success tend to decrease.

Another factor to consider alongside success rates is how long the clinic has been established. A particular clinic may have a great deal of experience in treating your particular problem, even if it's difficult to treat and has a low success rate, so it may be your best option. Mira remembers that it was tempting to go for a clinic which had a comparatively high success rate but,

'We had to look at places that were willing to treat the more difficult cases, like me, and if they do that then their figures might not be so high.'

Another thing to bear in mind when choosing a clinic, as Lena points out, is whether you're comfortable with the person in charge of your treatment.

'They may be a world expert but, if you don't find them friendly and approachable, they're not going to do you much good. You're putting yourself in the hands of this person and you may well be there a long time, so you've got to make sure you're happy to be there.'

COSTS

The cost of treatments also varies widely and this can affect your choice of clinic significantly. Whatever costs you are quoted before you begin treatment (whether or not some of your treatment is being funded by the NHS), make sure you ask:

- what is the full cost of each treatment cycle likely to be? (Each attempt at achieving a pregnancy is called a 'treatment cycle')
- exactly what do these costs cover? Do they cover all the tests the clinic will carry out? Will the drugs that are required be charged for separately?
- what possible extra charges might arise? Some clinics make additional charges for items such as initial assessments, follow-up consultations or embryo freezing and storage
- is there extra to pay for counselling at any stage?
- how much of the fee is refundable if a treatment cycle is abandoned at any stage for whatever reason?

The HFEA produces a *Patients' Guide* to all the centres in the UK which provide IVF and DI treatments; it contains a full list of questions that couples may like to consider asking any clinic before undergoing treatment. It is available free by calling the HFEA (see p. 278), or can be downloaded from the HFEA web site (see p. 290).

By asking at every stage about all aspects of the tests and treatment you are offered at a clinic, you will be better able to make an informed choice about the options that are open to you and what you should do next.

WILL THE CLINIC TREAT YOU?

The HFEA's *Code of Practice* makes it clear that, before agreeing to treat a particular couple, all licensed clinics must take into account the welfare of any potential child who may be born (or affected) as a result of the treatment. This means that clinics, before offering you any treatment, may ask you about:

- your age
- your medical history and that of your family
- how long you have been living together
- how many children you have in this or any other relationship
- whether you have any health problems which might influence a pregnancy or your ability to raise a child
- your commitment to having and bringing up a child or children
- the effects of the treatment on the couple's own health and welfare
- what effect a new baby or babies may have upon any child or children you already have

This may be done by interview, or you may be asked to complete a questionnaire before seeing the consultant. Occasionally there may be some information you do not wish to share with your partner (or want the clinic to pass back to your GP); remember that everything you tell a clinic is confidential, and the information cannot be shared with anyone without your permission.

Before agreeing to treat you, clinics will also consider:

- the needs of any child who may be born and your ability as prospective parents to meet those needs
- whether there is a risk of harm to the child or children who may be born

The approach may vary from one clinic to the next, but it is because of this legal obligation to consider 'the welfare of the child' that some clinics have refused treatment to single-sex couples and to potential parents who are HIV positive, for example. The final decision on whether or not to offer treatment to a particular person rests with the doctor concerned, and with the clinic's ethics committee if there is one. If you are refused treatment, the reasons should be explained to you fully, and advice given on what you could do next.

Most clinics have an upper age limit for women, although this limit varies. If you are over 40, or 45, you may have more difficulty in finding a clinic that is willing to treat you. Callie remembers having to 'fight' to get treatment at the age of 42, so if you are undertaking a similar battle you are not alone.

Remember, too, that as a matter of policy some private clinics don't offer treatment to single women or unmarried couples, so you cannot leap over all the hurdles which might be placed in your way simply by going private, although you might clear some.

HIV and hepatitis B and C testing

In line with the recommendations of the European Society of Human Reproduction and Embryology (ESHRE) and HFEA guidelines on 'the welfare of the child', most clinics now have a policy of testing all patients for HIV and hepatitis B and C before they undergo any treatment.

> **Confidentiality**
>
> You can, if you wish, keep your treatment an entirely private matter. Clinics cannot disclose information about your IVF or DI treatments, even to your GP, without your written consent. Passing on this information, except in very exceptional circumstances, is a criminal offence.

COUNSELLING AND SUPPORT

By law, all HFEA-licensed fertility treatment clinics must offer you the opportunity of talking to a counsellor before you begin any treatment. You don't have to take up this offer, but some clinics will insist on it before you can undergo certain treatments – for example, to make sure you have thought through all the implications before going ahead with IVF using donor eggs. Counselling can offer support, and is a therapeutic way of talking through your worries, about either the treatment itself or the effects of infertility on you as an individual and as a couple.

At what stage, if ever, you tell family and friends that you are having treatment is up to you. Who do you tell? How much do you tell them? There is more discussion of these issues in Chapter 10, because even if you begin treatment without feeling a need to tell anyone, there may come a point where your feelings change.

As you begin treatment, however, you may find the support of national self-help groups like CHILD or ISSUE (see pp. 278–9) of value. In addition, many hospitals and clinics have their own patient support groups.

What about adoption?

If you feel that adoption may be something you would consider, you need to examine your options even more carefully. Find out if your local social services department or adoption agencies have age restrictions: many won't accept couples as potential adoptive parents if one of you is over 35. If you're near that age now, you may have to decide whether to register your interest in adoption or go ahead with treatment. You won't be able to do both, as most agencies won't consider anyone for adoption if they are undergoing infertility treatment.

WHAT NEXT?

You have choices at every stage: to pursue treatment or reassess your objectives. Before undergoing any treatment you should consider carefully not only what is suitable but also what is acceptable for you as a couple. Some questions you may like to ask yourselves include:

- do we want to have any treatment?
- do we want to have the treatment that's on offer to us?
- what can our health authority offer us?
- can we afford private treatment?
- are we happy waiting a bit longer?

Your decision about whether to go ahead with treatment may largely depend on what is on offer on your area and whether you are eligible for and can afford private treatment, but it will also depend on what treatment you are offered. Some are less invasive and expensive than others. In Chapter 5 these treatments are looked at in detail.

5

The Experience of Treatment

Many fertility treatments put great stress on the couple, especially the woman, who is usually the focus of the medical interventions. You may need to make several visits to the clinic or to your GP for injections, blood tests, scans, monitoring and so forth. Make sure you know the practicalities of what is involved before you go ahead. You should also get a clear picture of how likely the treatment is to help you, and what side-effects you may experience. Always ask any questions which you consider important because treatment for infertility is an uncertain process at best, so the more you understand, the better.

The treatments looked at in this chapter are:

- *hormone treatments*: stimulation of ovulation may be done on its own or combined with other treatments like IUI (intrauterine insemination) or in vitro fertilisation (IVF)
- *surgery*: this is sometimes suggested to unblock the fallopian tubes or for blockages in the male reproductive system
- *artificial insemination/IUI*
- *IVF*: including the combination of IVF with micromanipulation techniques
- *GIFT (gamete intrafallopian transfer)*

In addition, there is some information about frozen embryos, which may be created as part of an IVF or GIFT cycle.

You may find that you move from one treatment to another, and some treatments will be synchronised: for example, a woman may take a course of hormones for a few months before the couple go on to try IUI.

HORMONE TREATMENTS

While men are sometimes given hormone treatment to improve sperm counts if their own levels of pituitary hormones are low, a 'front-line therapy' for many couples is a course of drugs to help stimulate and regularise ovulation.

Clomiphene citrate (brand names: Clomid and Serophene) is a synthetic drug taken in tablet form, and is often the first drug that's tried if you have irregular ovulation resulting from hormonal imbalances. It's usually taken daily between Days 2 and 6 of your cycle, with the aim of stimulating the ovaries into ovulation. The drug works because it is similar in structure to oestrogen and so blocks the oestrogen receptors in the brain: the brain then interprets this as a lack of oestrogen and triggers the pituitary to release more FSH and LH, the hormones responsible for egg development and ovulation. The lowest dose given is 50mg, although your doctor may increase this (occasionally up to 200mg) if lower doses don't work (i.e. make you ovulate) within a couple of months. If it doesn't seem to be working, your doctor can check by testing your hormone levels with a blood test around Day 21 or checking your ovaries with an ultrasound scan in mid-cycle to see if any follicles are developing.

For many women, a course of clomiphene does seem like a miracle cure. Amy found then such a miracle that she didn't even need to take them.

'I came home from the chemist with that little packet of pills clutched in my hand. I felt so good. After all those months of charting, of desperation, my GP was taking my concerns seriously and I had the answer to all my problems right here in my hand. I was even looking forward to my next cycle starting, as I knew everything would be

different this time. So I went home from the doctor's with a happy heart . . . and if I didn't conceive that night, I conceived the next. I never took a single pill and the next cycle never started because I was already pregnant.'

Few of us are quite that lucky, but Cora felt lucky, too:

'We'd heard so many stories about how long it took some people to conceive that we were geared up for years of treatment if necessary. As it turned out, I wasn't ovulating, was prescribed Clomid, and was pregnant within three months. All I needed was a kick-start.'

Perhaps because they do help so many women, these drugs can be invested with a huge amount of hope. Ruth has been through two cycles of stimulation with no happy result, and it's making her feel despondent:

'I'm worried we're in for a big battle ahead and this is only just the start.'

Jayne says,

'My GP diagnosed a mild ovulation problem and prescribed me Clomid. He said, "You'll be pregnant within three months and the next time we see you, it'll be at the antenatal clinic." I believed him. But I was on Clomid for ten cycles and didn't get pregnant, so was advised to move on to fertility injections.'

Gilli also had to come to terms with disappointment:

'When I was given my first treatment, in the form of hormone tablets, I thought this was the magic I had been waiting for, particularly when I was told that these tablets were successful for 80 per cent of women. I couldn't believe that I wouldn't be in that group, but I wasn't. I was one of the other 20 per cent.'

Taking a course of clomiphene may bring certain side-effects, although it is sincerely hoped that the main side-effect you will experience is pregnancy. However, because your ovaries are stimulated, you run the risk of producing more than one egg in each cycle, which can result in you becoming pregnant with twins (or, rarely, more). While a multiple pregnancy seems to occur for only about one in 15 women who conceive while taking clomiphene, it's something you need to be aware of.

There are less pleasant side-effects, too. Some women on clomiphene find that it makes them irritable and restless and gives them headaches. Others get some breast tenderness, mild abdominal discomfort or hot flushes. A few get more severe side-effects, such as nausea and vomiting, pain or vision difficulties, in which case they should stop taking the tablets immediately.

If you have been keeping BBT charts, you may find that drugs to stimulate ovulation cause a change of pattern, making it even more difficult to know if or when you are ovulating. Jo says,

'I conceived on Clomid and was convinced I wouldn't as my temperature hadn't risen at all. It just hovered around the same mark and I had no idea whether we'd had sex at the right time or not.'

High doses of clomiphene can interfere with your body's natural cervical mucus changes, too, but, as Helen says,

'If you're having sex every two or three days in the middle two weeks of your cycle, you're bound to hit the right time.'

However, many women find that one of the main advantages of clomiphene is that it regulates their periods, which makes it easier to know when ovulation is likely to be, and therefore when to have sex . . . but, as ever, timing sex to both partner's desires is still not easy. Gilli recalls:

'There was so much pressure on both of us – performing at the right time, waiting to see if the treatment had worked, and trying to get ourselves back on an even keel each time that it hadn't.'

Zoë has been trying to conceive for about two years, and has been on Clomid for nearly nine months.

'It hasn't worked and I now want to stop taking it because I've read of the risks, including cancer. Now I have to go back to my GP and see where that leaves us.'

Zoë is right: several studies have suggested that women taking drugs to stimulate their ovaries (including Clomid, but also some of the injectible hormones) are at an increased risk of ovarian cancer. While research into this is still continuing, it is nevertheless recommended by the Committee on the Safety of Medicine that you should normally only use clomiphene for six cycles. Although there are stories about women who have finally conceived after two years on Clomid, do remember that if it hasn't worked for you after six cycles, the chances are it isn't ever going to work. Most women whom the drug can help will have conceived by then. Unfortunately, even while it stimulates many women to ovulate, the effect that Clomid can have on the cervical mucus can make it more difficult for sperm to penetrate, so for this reason it may not work for you.

If the tablets don't kick your system into action, you may be advised to move on to a course of injections designed to stimulate the ovaries, which is not a pleasant prospect if you hate needles. Rosemary says,

'I couldn't stand the thought of someone sticking a needle in my body every day for God knows how many days. I thought I'd ask Richard to do it, but he just turned white.'

The injections which you may be prescribed, sometimes in conjunction with the tablets, will probably be one of the following:

- hMG (human menopausal gonadotrophin, which is a mixture of LH and FSH, in drugs such as Pergonal). This is an intra-muscular injection (which needs a long needle), given over several days in the first half of your cycle. It directly stimulates the ovaries to produce and mature eggs
- FSH (in drugs such as Metrodin HP). Purified FSH can be given by subcutaneous injection (which only needs a short needle and is much less painful) and acts directly to stimulate the follicles
- hCG (human chorionic gonadotrophin). This is given by your doctor in one injection at the right point in your cycle and helps to ensure that the developing egg(s) will be released. It triggers ovulation the way LH does in a natural cycle

Some women tolerate, as well as respond to, certain drugs better than others. Genetically engineered FSH (in brands such as Gonal-F) is now available, which is even purer and can cause less of an adverse reaction, but it is more expensive.

Where do the drugs come from?

The original hormones used in fertility treatment were derived from the urine of menopausal women. Women in this age group produce high levels of FSH with some LH in the form of hMG (human menopausal gonadotrophin), and this hormone was extracted and marketed under various names including Pergonal and Humegon. However, demand for these 'urinary' hormones increased as more and more couples wanted to make use of techniques like IVF and ICSI, so they became in very short supply. Drug manufacturers therefore developed recombinant FSH produced by genetic engineering – hamster cells are altered genetically to produce human FSH.

An alternative treatment involves the use of GnRH. Normally, GnRH stimulates the release of LH and FSH from the pituitary by sending out small chemical messengers at regular intervals. This natural process can be imitated by attaching a small pump to your upper arm with a tiny tube going into one of your veins. Small pulses of GnRH are then pumped into your body over several days.

Ask your doctor which drug or combination of drugs he wants to put you on and why. Some are more suitable for women with polycystic ovaries, for example, and others may have to be avoided if you have a known allergy – Metrodin HP contains lactose, for instance. Ask about the side-effects to look out for (and there are always some, even if you only feel them mildly) before you begin taking them.

Ovarian hyperstimulation syndrome

Sometimes, despite careful monitoring, a woman's ovaries respond very strongly to the injected drugs given to coax them into producing a larger number of eggs than usual and begin to swell. This may result in ovarian hyperstimulation syndrome, which can result in a range of symptoms including mild to severe abdominal pain, vomiting, nausea, dizziness, dehydration and headaches. For those experiencing mild symptoms, drinking plenty of fluids, resting and taking painkillers will probably be enough. Severe cases require admission to hospital for treatment and bed rest. Clinics will give you an emergency number to ring if you are worried you are experiencing hyperstimulation, because if it is left untreated it becomes very dangerous indeed.

There is also the risk, when you move on to the 'heavy-duty hormone injections', that your ovaries will over-respond and produce too many eggs. Because ovarian hyperstimulation can cause complications, you will be carefully monitored through ultrasound scans and blood tests to check the development of the follicles in your ovaries. If it becomes clear that too many eggs are developing, you will be advised to avoid sex during that cycle because of the risks of a high-order multiple pregnancy.

Ovulation stimulation can feel like it's going to be the big breakthrough, but it doesn't work for everyone. Gilli found that her body did not react predictably to the hormone injections and her periods became more and more erratic.

'Life was so cruel . . . Every time one was late, I would think, "This is it" and do another pregnancy test, sometimes two or three, unable to believe that my body could be doing this to me.'

Jayne agrees:

'You go through so much – the scans and the blood tests and the build-up to each treatment – that it's very stressful and it's heartbreaking when each cycle fails.'

Ovulation stimulation

Advantages
- relatively non-intrusive
- has a relatively high success rate
- Clomid is often available on prescription from your GP

Disadvantages
- side-effects
- long-term health risks associated with over six months' usage of any dosage
- high doses of clomiphene may increase the risk of miscarriage

SURGERY

Nobody undertakes surgery lightly, and for many couples these days techniques such as IVF and ICSI are a preferred option if this treatment is available through their health authority or they can afford it themselves. However, surgery does have benefits and may well be the first (or only) treatment you are offered by your health authority.

Men may be recommended surgery if, because of injury, infection, congenital abnormality or previous surgery such as a vasectomy, the ducts through which the sperm travels have become blocked. Sometimes it is suggested that a man has surgery to remove a varicocoele (swollen vein) if it may be interfering with sperm production or movement; this can be done under local anaesthetic.

Surgery may be recommended if you have endometriosis: it may be possible to remove some of the cells with a laser via a laparoscopy, or you may need more extensive surgery. It may also be advised if you have adhesions or fibroids within your uterus, or to open a narrow or scarred cervix. It is sometimes also needed to treat polycystic ovaries.

As one of the most common reasons for a woman being unable to conceive is blocked fallopian tubes, you may be offered surgery to unblock them if you are in this category. Surgery can often be very successful in removing adhesions and endometriosis where this affects the tubes, although the chances of success decrease the greater the blockage or the damage, and a few women who undergo surgery find that their tubes become blocked again. If the surgery can be done through a laparoscopy, a large incision in your abdomen will be avoided. Nevertheless, surgery always involves the risks and side-effects associated with a general anaesthetic and will mean that you need to stay in hospital for a few days, and will probably need several weeks to recover fully.

One of the greatest advantages of surgery is that, if it works, it means that you will be able to go on and have a 'spontaneous' conception, without the need for further treatment.

Lara was offered surgery to repair a blocked fallopian tube but decided to go for IVF instead.

'I was worried that the abdominal surgery might just bring further adhesions, and could actually lower our chances. IVF seemed to offer more hope.'

Her concerns are understandable: the surgery itself may cause the development of adhesions, which can reduce your fertility, although you will be given antibiotics and anti-inflammatory drugs to reduce the risk of this happening. Also, the risk of an ectopic pregnancy is higher after you have had tubal surgery because, if the adhesions or endometriosis return, this can prevent a developing embryo from reaching the uterus and it becomes lodged in the tube instead. If you do miss a period after tubal surgery, let your doctor know immediately so that you can have an early ultrasound scan to check that the embryo has implanted where it should.

Some recent studies[4] have shown that tube blockage does affect the success rate of IVF. If the blockage causes a hydrosalpinx, where the follicular fluid builds up, this fluid seems to leak into the uterus and lower the chances of an embryo implanting. This is something you need to take into account if your fallopian tubes are blocked.

You may find that you are offered a relatively new surgical treatment, in which a catheter is passed through your cervix and into your uterus and dye is injected through the catheter into the tubes to show the source of the blockage (as in an HSG, as described on p. 70). Once the point of the blockage can be seen, a thin wire is passed down the tube to unblock it. You don't need a general anaesthetic for this procedure, so it carries fewer risks.

Surgery

Advantages
- if it works it can be the ultimate cure, restoring your fertility permanently
- surgery is funded by many health authorities
- it is more widely available than many assisted conception techniques

Disadvantages
- side-effects associated with general anaesthesia
- it can take you a long time to recover
- small risk of further adhesions or blockages developing as a result of the operation itself
- it leaves you in an uncertain state for many months as you wait and wonder whether the treatment has worked

New hope for infertile men?

Recently, surgical techniques have been developed which offer real hope to men with low sperm counts, or who are producing sperm whose passage through the epididymis is blocked so that none appears in the semen. In the past, the only chance of a couple being able to conceive would have been by using donor sperm. The new techniques allow the sperm to be surgically extracted, after which it can be used in IVF treatment. They can also help men who have undergone a vasectomy reversal which has failed. The various techniques are as follows:

- *micro-epididymal sperm aspiration (MESA)*: sperm are collected directly from the epididymis
- *percutaneous sperm aspiration (PESA)*: in this variation, a local anaesthetic is used and a needle is inserted through the skin of the testicle to extract sperm from the epididymis

- *testicular sperm extraction (TESE)*: sperm are collected directly from the testicles

One thought: these treatments, while new, and promising a high success rate, are expensive.

ARTIFICIAL INSEMINATION/ INTRAUTERINE INSEMINATION

Artificial insemination (AI) is a comparatively simple method of assisted conception. It involves placing the semen either at the top of the vagina or into the cervix. It has a long history – there are old stories of women inseminating themselves using a straw – and it seems much less high-tech than some other methods of assisted conception. As it gets sperm past the vagina, AI can help couples where the man's sperm may be killed off by the acidic secretions, and also those couples who are unable to have sexual intercourse because of injury, disability or difficulties such as premature ejaculation.

The insemination itself is straightforward. The doctor or nurse inserts a fine plastic tube into the woman's vagina through which the sperm is then placed into the mucus in the cervix. With intrauterine insemination (IUI), semen (which has been 'washed' and treated to retrieve the best-quality motile sperm) is introduced directly into the woman's uterus at around the time of ovulation, with the aim of helping the sperm get closer to the site of fertilisation. You rest for a short time afterwards, and then carry on life as normal. Either the husband's (or partner's) sperm or donor sperm is used. The use of donor sperm is covered in more detail in Chapter 6.

Because successful AI/IUI depends on the ability of sperm to fertilise an egg, a man will need to be producing enough normal sperm in reasonable numbers, although the procedure can help in cases where the motility of the sperm has been causing problems. Obviously, it can also only help couples in which the woman is ovulating and has open fallopian tubes. Although it is a relatively straightforward procedure, success is not guaranteed, especially when the woman is over 35.

Insemination is carried out during the most fertile part of the woman's cycle, sometimes on two or three days in a row. Some clinics do AI/IUI alone, without chemical regulation of the woman's ovaries; instead they rely on BBT charts, cervical mucus changes, OPKs and sometimes ultrasound scans to ensure that insemination coincides with the optimum pre-ovulation days. In other cases insemination is carried out in conjunction with ovarian stimulation, for example a course of clomiphene, to ensure egg development and ovulation. This seems to produce better results – success rates can reach 30 per cent.

Alison found the routine for getting her body ready for AI demanding.

'Every day I had to go for injections or to have blood taken or a scan. We're lucky – we only live an hour's drive away from the clinic. Some couples were coming from much further away for treatment.'

Robin and Tracy found their experience demoralising:

'The treatment involved Tracy consuming large quantities of tablets and having to visit the local maternity hospital for a set of unnecessarily painful injections. Unfortunately, those administering them seemed unable to appreciate that Tracy, at just over six stone, didn't have a lot of substance in which to take an intra-muscular injection.'

David found the experience of producing the semen necessary for AI a very degrading moment.

'I was shown into this tiny room with a single bed with just a mattress, no sheets, a minute washbasin. It didn't seem the right environment to be starting a child, but it had to be done. I stood there and thought, "If I can't do this, we've got a big problem . . ." so it had to be done.'

Sharon and Alex chose to 'collect' the semen necessary for their AI in a special non-spermicidal condom during intercourse.

'We were so uncomfortable with the idea of Alex masturbating over some dirty pictures that we decided we would do it this way, even though we were warned that what we brought along might not be good enough. It was one way to make the whole thing less clinical.'

Robin too had trouble with his contribution to the process:

'The specimen that I managed to produce was, to say the least, diminutive. Then I got stuck in a traffic jam while rushing to the hospital, with my seminal fluids safely deposited back where they came from, in my trousers, but this time in a jar wrapped in cotton wool, silver foil and held together with a sock in an attempt to keep it alive. All so that it could be "washed and percolated", or, in other words, the good bits extracted and made ready to be injected into Tracy's uterus at the appropriate time the next day. However poor my sample was, an amount for injection was produced and we went ahead.'

Robin and Tracy found that their troubles continued:

'The next problem was the doctor, whom we had never met, who walked into the room, didn't introduce himself and proceeded to perform the attempted IUI in a manner akin to a bull in a china shop. Our first attempt failed, and we wanted to make sure that next time we would know who was going to be performing the procedure and that it would be completed with a great deal more dignity. They obliged.'

Some women do find the IUI procedure uncomfortable, even when done with care, especially if the cervix is far back or tilted at an 'awkward' angle. Diane says,

'I felt more pressure than anything, like I needed a wee. The nurse said it was because the catheter had got a good seal on my cervix. As soon as she took it out I felt better, though a bit tender.'

Cathy found it much, much easier than she had expected.

'I'd heard some horror stories and spent the night before really worrying about what I was letting myself in for. I did feel uncomfortable at one point, when they were opening the cervix and it felt like stretching. But when I asked the doctor how much longer it was going to take, he said it was already over and they were taking the catheter out. It was over before I knew it.'

Gail found it more uncomfortable:

'It did hurt when they were opening my cervix, and they needed to use metal clips to hold the uterus open. I also had cramps when they did the insemination, which the nurse said was not unusual – your uterus isn't used to having liquid injected into it.'

Amber, even though AI worked for her, was left with lingering disappointment about the clinical process:

'Somehow, this wasn't the mystical moment of conception I'd always imagined. There was a nurse there I'd never met before, and I felt like something from an animal husbandry class. I know these feelings will go when the baby arrives, but they're here now.'

Robin and Tracy found that IUI didn't work for them, but something else did:

'Unfortunately, our second attempt failed to produce any eggs and the third was unsuccessful because my sperm count was too low. So about three weeks after our third failed programme, we were summoned to the consultant's inner sanctum and told very sympathetically that, due to my

low sperm production, further attempts at IUI would be pointless. They would refer us on for IVF but couldn't say how long this would take, irrespective of our circumstances. We went home feeling rather depressed, but at the same time relieved that there was further help and that all we had to do was wait. We decided that the best thing to do was to forget all our worries and go and enjoy some stress-free lovemaking. If our calculations are correct, Tracy conceived that day. We now have a beautiful baby boy.'

IVF

You may be offered IVF if you have damaged or blocked fallopian tubes, perhaps through scarring or endometriosis, and the chances of repairing them through microsurgery aren't good. It can also help couples where the man has a low sperm count or where the sperm don't move forward very well and so may never reach the egg without assistance. In addition, couples whose infertility is caused by immunological factors – the presence of antibodies in the semen or cervical mucus – can find that IVF bypasses this problem. And, of course, it does offer a chance of conceiving to couples whose infertility lies in the category of 'unexplained.'

Considering IVF

Before beginning any IVF treatment, the clinic must obtain your written 'informed' consent. This means that you must have been given:

- all the information you need about the process of treatment
- the chance to discuss any concerns you may have with staff at the clinic
- the opportunity to talk to a counsellor
- time to think about your decision

You will also be asked (as will donors) for written consent to the use and storage of sperm, eggs and any resultant embryos, which can then only be used in the way that you have decided. Take the time to read through your consent forms carefully and ask as many questions as you like about anything you do not understand. Signing the consent form in itself does not commit you to anything: you are free to change your mind at any time.

Before going ahead, Eilish read up as much as she could about the treatment and its long-term effects:

'I read some studies which showed that there was possibly an increased risk of ovarian cancer in women who had had IVF treatment, but I felt that this, and some other studies, were inconclusive. Who's to say these women weren't predisposed to it anyway, because of their problems in conceiving? But I wanted as much information as possible, so I knew what the risks might be to my health and my body.'

What happens?

In IVF, eggs are gathered from the woman's ovaries and mixed with sperm. The fertilised egg (or embryo) is then transferred to the woman's uterus. 'In vitro' comes from the Latin, meaning literally 'in glass', which refers to the glass container in the laboratory where fertilisation takes place. This is usually a flat Petri dish, though in the popular consciousness the 'glass vessel' has become a test tube – hence the term 'test-tube babies'.

While this sounds reasonably straightforward, it is in fact a complex, stressful and demanding process, especially for the woman. A single treatment cycle (from beginning to take the necessary drugs to doing a pregnancy test) can take between six weeks and two months, and will include phases when you have to have injections every day, regular ultrasound monitoring, and surgery carried out at exactly the right time. A powerful message from couples who have been through IVF is not to underestimate what will be required of you, in terms of both physical commitment and stress and the emotional rollercoaster you are climbing aboard. The more information you can get from your clinic, your support group and other couples before you begin, the better.

What is a 'treatment cycle'?

In IVF using 'fresh' embryos (ones that haven't been frozen), a cycle begins when the woman starts on the drugs which aim to produce several eggs in her ovaries (a stimulated cycle). If these drugs aren't used (an unstimulated or 'natural' cycle), a cycle is deemed to have started with the attempt to collect eggs.

In IVF using embryos that have been frozen, a cycle begins with the removal of the embryos from storage. Not all embryos survive the thawing process, so that cycle may never reach embryo transfer stage.

Cultivating the eggs

Normally, a woman will produce only one egg in each menstrual cycle. However, because your chances of getting pregnant through IVF are much higher if more than one embryo is replaced, the woman's ovaries are usually stimulated so that several eggs mature. This has the advantage of increasing your chances of pregnancy, but does mean that you are subjecting your body to some very powerful medication.

A variety of drugs are used, and the doctor treating you will decide what will be most appropriate in your case according to a range of factors including your age and the levels of hormones you normally produce. In addition, how many days you stay on each drug and the dosages you need will vary, depending on how your body is responding to treatment. No two women will respond in the same way, which is one reason you will be so closely monitored throughout. If the side-effects become intolerable or you turn out to be allergic to one brand of drug, there are alternatives.

You normally need to start taking the drugs in advance of the start of your cycle, or on the first day of your period. First of all, to suppress your own pituitary system you will need to take drugs such as Synarel, Buserelin or Zoladex, either in the form of a nasal spray or as an injection. You need to sniff the nasal spray every four hours (though you can omit the one in the middle of the night) or have the injections twice a day, morning and evening. This phase of the treatment lasts about 21 days. The drugs have the effect of putting your body into a temporary menopause, along with all the side-effects you might expect: hot flushes, mood swings and irregular bleeding . . .

Around Day 14 of your cycle, you will have a blood test and scan at your clinic to check that your ovaries have, in fact, been suppressed. If not, you'll need to continue with the drugs and return at a later date. If they have been suppressed, you can now begin the drugs that will stimulate egg production. These are usually injections of hMG, which is a mixture of LH and FSH (drugs such as Pergonal), or FSH (in drugs such as Metrodin). Or you may be given a combination of tablets (clomiphene) and injections.

The clinic staff can show your partner how to give you the injections. While this can cut down the number of visits you have to make to the clinic, not all couples take up this offer. Some injections are done subcutaneously, into the skin, which only requires a short needle, while others have to be done into the muscle, with a longer needle, which can be more painful (though many women say the anticipation of the injection is worse than the injection itself). Some women experience side-effects such as abdominal bloating, rashes, more mood swings and aching muscles. Others find that they gain weight due to increased salt and water retention in their bodies. You can expect to be on these injections for around 12 days (and you'll still be taking your suppression sniffs to prevent you ovulating before the egg collection), but this will vary according to the way you respond.

Clinics must carefully monitor the way your ovaries are responding to the treatment, not least because of the risk of overstimulation. To do so they use ultrasound scanning (usually three or four scans in each treatment cycle), which shows the size and number of developing follicles. While the eggs are maturing, the follicles produce a hormone called oestradiol. Some women are also asked to come in for blood tests to check their oestradiol levels, which can indicate how the eggs are developing, so you may find yourself attending the IVF clinic frequently during this stage.

Transport IVF

Some clinics offer a service called 'transport IVF'. This means that tests, ovulation treatment and egg retrieval are carried out in a centre near the couple's home, which is not necessarily HFEA-licensed as these treatments don't need a licence. The eggs are then transported in an incubator to a licensed IVF unit, and it's here that fertilisation and embryo transfer take place. This arrangement can reduce the stress of frequent long journeys for women who don't live near an IVF clinic. You will be given full information about the procedure, be offered counselling and be asked for your written consent to treatment before the egg retrieval procedure is begun, just as you would be if your entire treatment was taking place in an HFEA-licensed clinic.

How does it feel?

The innocuous little warning on some leaflets that the medication you are taking to stimulate your ovaries can cause 'mood swings' proves to be a severe understatement for some women. Says Barbara,

'It turns me into a witch, No one dares come near me.'

Hannah found it was more like

'pre-menstrual tension, tetchiness and depression, spread over several weeks instead of a couple of days'.

Karen found that one of the most difficult parts of the ordeal was 'getting up at the crack of dawn to travel to the clinic nearly every day' for her injections. Even if you have these at your GP practice, or your partner learns how to give them to you, you will still need to go to the clinic for monitoring how the eggs are developing.

Eilish found that she lost a sense of control very early in the process:

'One of the hardest things for me to come to terms with was the idea that my own natural cycle was being suppressed and all these artificial hormones were taking it over, stimulating my ovaries above and beyond what they would normally do. I felt like I was entirely at someone's else's mercy, especially as I knew things didn't always work out and I might not develop any follicles, or develop too many.'

These things do happen to some women, or they may produce follicles which are then found not to contain any eggs.

Deanne says,

'The thing about IVF that I found hardest to come to terms with is that it's not the exact science I thought it was. In my first two cycles I overstimulated, and I also needed to take hormones to thicken the lining of the womb, and they just couldn't get the balance of everything right.'

Tina experienced this too:

'The first cycle they gave me really low levels of drugs to avoid hyperstimulation, and I didn't produce any eggs at all. The next, only two.'

Getting the balance of drugs right for each individual can take a few cycles, so don't lose hope if your first treatment cycle ends because the drugs aren't working yet for you. It doesn't mean that future cycles won't be successful; in fact your consultant will now have a better idea of how your body responds to the various drugs, so next time the medication can be better adapted to your responses. However, any abandoned treatment cycle isn't good news if you are paying for treatment yourselves and you can only afford a limited number of cycles in the first place, although your clinic will probably give you a partial refund for an abandoned attempt.

Another thing many women have problems coming to terms with is the fact that the process seems so divorced from what they're trying to achieve – sniffing powerful hormones is very far removed from cuddling a baby. Caroline, on her third cycle of IVF, has to remind herself how strange everything really is when she has become so used to it.

'I sometimes think, when Paul is giving me one of the injections, "How did we ever get to this?" It's alarming, sometimes, what can come to seem second nature.' Liam, too, found that going with Colleen for ultrasound monitoring to check the developing follicles left him with an overwhelming sense of 'How did we get here?' If you find yourselves asking each other that, you won't be the first. Sometimes, because of all these pressures, couples themselves ask for a break in the treatment.

Abandoned cycles

In around 18 per cent of cases a treatment cycle has to be abandoned before egg collection takes place. This could happen because you don't produce enough follicles or because they grow very poorly. Low levels of oestradiol can indicate that the eggs aren't developing properly. Sometimes ovarian hyperstimulation means the treatment has to be cancelled. If any of these things happen to you, the cycle will be abandoned. You will be given advice on how long it might be best to wait before starting another, depending on what has happened to you.

Egg collection/retrieval

Exactly when egg collection is done depends on how your ovaries respond to the stimulation of the drugs you are given. It takes place when the ultrasound scan shows that you have a sufficient number of large follicles (18mm or more in size). You will have an intramuscular injection of hCG (Profasi/Pregnyl) very late at night. This injection gives the eggs their last 'push' towards maturity. Ovulation would normally occur between 37 and 40 hours after this injection, so the egg collection is therefore scheduled to take place (in the daytime) just before the follicles burst.

Although it is a relatively quick and painless procedure, it is stressful. Many women report worrying dreams about egg collections going wrong, perhaps not unexpectedly when so much depends on it. Roseanne says,

'The night before I dreamt they were taking out each of the eggs and squashing them. Not deliberately, – they just got squashed in the tube. I watched as one after the other disappeared and there didn't seem to be anything I could do. Needless to say, when I turned up at the hospital the next day I was shaking like a leaf.'

Before egg collection begins, the man needs to produce his semen sample. Although much of the focus in IVF is on the woman, the man comes under stress, too. Richard admits he did not enjoy having to go to a hospital room and masturbate while his partner was getting prepared for theatre. Mike, too, felt this part of the process was very clinical.

'The clinic information said something like, "We have a private room for the production of semen samples," which we laughed about beforehand as where else would they expect you to do it? And there was all this business about, "We ask you to refrain from sexual intercourse for two or three days beforehand in order to produce the optimum ejaculate." Well, of course, once you're in this private room, which is just a room full of dirty magazines, there's a lot of pressure on you to produce this "optimum ejaculate" because you know they're waiting outside the door to whisk it away.'

Matt found that

'I had done it so many times before at the hospital for one test or another that I had sort of got used to it. I looked on it as something that had to be done – not anything special. But there's very few fathers who can remember the night their children were conceived as something particularly special or memorable, so it didn't matter overmuch.'

The semen is assessed and, if it's of good enough quality, the sperm are 'washed' in preparation for fertilisation. Occasionally the semen sample is not deemed adequate and the man has to be prevailed upon to produce another one.

The eggs are usually collected using a fine, hollow needle guided by ultrasound. You will be given a light sedative, so you shouldn't feel any pain and you may not remember much about it afterwards, though you can watch the images on the ultrasound screen if you're awake enough. The doctor will put a small probe into your vagina, which guides the needle into each ovary, and the fluid containing the egg is sucked from each of the mature follicles through the needle. The contents of each follicle are examined under a microscope to see if an egg is present. Callie remembers hearing someone shout 'Egg' from a far corner of the room from time to time. Although most clinics prefer to use a local anaesthetic so the procedure can be done on an outpatient day care basis, occasionally egg collection is done under a general anaesthetic via laparoscopy or using an abdominal needle.

Roseanne recalls,

'I was given a general anaesthetic for mine, though I know that some clinics give you a local. It was very quick and easy, about 20 minutes. I was a bit crampy for a few hours, but that went away before long.'

For Jana, however, it was more uncomfortable:

'I found it difficult. I was given some light sedation but even so it wasn't pleasant. At least it was over pretty quickly.'

Liam, though he wasn't the one involved in the procedure, found it sparked strong feelings in him.

'I felt really guilty. We only need IVF because I have such a low sperm count, and I know that Colleen didn't have this in mind when she said "For better or for worse." I'm the one with the problem, but she's the one lying on the table while they poke about inside her with a needle.'

The clinic will tell you how many eggs they managed to collect. After a short rest, you'll be able to go home. Some women do feel uncomfortable after egg collection, and sensations of bloating and pain may take a few hours to fade, but these are probably minor compared to what is going on in your mind. For now that they've been collected, what's happening to the eggs?

From egg to embryo

As soon as the eggs are extracted, they're put into a nutrient medium and both the eggs and the sperm are then cultured (usually overnight) in an incubator. The next day, they'll be observed through a microscope to see if fertilisation has occurred. If it has, then 24 hours later cell division will have started and the 'pre-embryo' might now have two or four cells. The embryos will be checked by an embryologist to make sure that they're developing normally and, if all is well, embryo transfer can now take place. Roseanne found this waiting time difficult:

'When I was waiting to find out how many fertilised, and then how they were developing, that was very nerve-racking – and there was absolutely nothing you could do, either, which was worse.'

You will be given a prescription for progesterone, which will be needed to provide hormonal support to any potential pregnancy. The progesterone will come either as pessaries (Cyclogest) which need to be inserted into your vagina twice a day, or injections, or you may be given injections of hCG.

If you're lucky, you'll get a call from the clinic to report on the good progress of your embryos and find yourself returning there 48 hours after egg collection, this time for the transfer.

Occasionally no eggs will fertilise at all. This generally happens when there has been a problem with the man's sperm, but it sometimes occurs even when everything appears normal. However, most couples will find that the eggs do fertilise and, of those, some will develop into embryos.

Transfer

When you come in for transfer, you'll be advised on how your embryos have developed and, if there are several of good quality, whether you want to have two or three transferred. To reduce the risk of a multiple pregnancy, the law states that no more than three embryos can be replaced. Many clinics recommend transferring two if the woman is under 30 years old, because this gives a good chance of success while reducing the risks of a multiple birth. The doctor will advise you in making the choice right for you and your circumstances.

Even transferring two means that you run the risk of having twins or more ('or more' because embryos have been known to split after transfer and to produce triplets). The idea of a multiple pregnancy may seem delightful when you've come this far in your struggle to have children at all, but it carries real risks, both for the woman and for the babies she is carrying: you are more likely to have blood pressure problems, premature birth and poor growth rates. However, the final decision on whether to transfer two or three embryos is yours, so this is something to which you need to give careful consideration beforehand, however remote a possibility it seems. It's all too easy to sidestep this important issue. Roseanne says,

'My main concern was getting pregnant. I thought I'd worry about anything else later.'

Often, however, the counting game goes the other way. Rachel had seven eggs collected, five of which fertilised, out of which just two developed into four-celled embryos by transfer stage.

'I had those two transferred and the other three were left to perish, because I was told they weren't of good enough quality to survive the freezing process. I was very sad about that, because I had looked on all five as potential children.'

Out of the two embryos transferred, one implanted and Rachel gave birth to a daughter,

'But I still have the memory of those other possible babies. When you invest everything with such significance, you don't just forget what might have been.'

How do they choose the embryos?

As a maximum of only three embryos can be transferred, sometimes a choice has to be made as to the 'best' to transfer. Many couples wonder how one embryo is judged over another in this 'beauty contest' in the laboratory dish.

The embryologist will examine the developing embryos and check for the symmetry of the cells, how much fragmentation there is, and how fast and well the embryos are growing. If an embryo has developed to the four-cell stage 38 hours after fertilisation, for example, this is an excellent indication. However, sometimes even the most promising embryos do not implant, and conversely every embryologist in the world can tell stories of deciding to transfer an unpromising embryo in the absence of any others, only to see it develop into a healthy and beautiful child. Nature does not deal in statistical absolutes, and although the embryologists will make the best choices they can, don't despair completely if you are initially told that your embryos are 'poor-quality'.

If you're lucky enough to have 'spare' embryos of good quality (only very high-quality ones will withstand cryopreservation), these can be frozen and stored ready to be replaced in a future treatment cycle – though not even all of these will make it through the freezing and thawing process. (There is more about the dilemmas posed by embryo freezing on p. 139.)

Transfer is usually straightforward. The embryos, together with a tiny amount of culture fluid, are put into a catheter and this is placed in your uterus through the cervix. Roseanne says,

'It was very easy. I didn't need an anaesthetic and the transfer itself was very quick. I just had to lie there for an hour afterwards and then they sent me home.'

If you're lucky, you'll be shown your embryos on a monitor before the transfer takes place. Barbara found this 'one of the most rewarding experiences of my life', as many couples do.

'They looked so perfect, so tiny, it was hard not to imagine a little child growing from each of them. I tried hard not to let my mind go too far down that path, because I knew it would just make everything harder to deal with if none of them implanted, but I didn't regret that moment.'

The wait

Of all the stages of any assisted conception treatment, this is perhaps the hardest. It will be about two weeks before you can have a pregnancy test, though for many couples it feels like several years. You will be advised to 'carry on as normal' once you get home, and some women manage to do so. More than one study has shown that the amount of physical activity you undertake doesn't affect the chances of implantation, but this won't stop many women thinking that it might. Barbara says,

'They say you don't need to rest in bed, but I felt like I wanted to, so I stayed in bed for the next couple of days. Then the dreaded wait began.'

Sara found the interval after embryo transfer 'agonising'.

'It really was two weeks of agonising, as well.'

The length of time may vary – in some clinics the pregnancy test can be done at 11 days following embryo transfer – but even so it takes its toll. Alison recalls,

'It was the longest two weeks of my life. They tell you to keep yourself busy but not to do anything – and don't think about it, either.'

Roseanne, too, found the wait very stressful:

'I was very emotional all the time, and could hardly think about anything else, worrying it wasn't going to work, knowing it wasn't going to work, and just thrown into terrible despair when it didn't work.'

After two weeks, if your period hasn't started you can go back to the clinic for a blood test to check the levels of the pregnancy hormone beta hCG – and you often get the results the same day. If the levels are high, you're pregnant. If the test is negative, you'll find that your period usually starts within a couple of days. Sometimes the progesterone pessaries themselves seem to 'hold off' menstruation, making your period later than normal, giving you time to get your hopes up . . . just in time for them to be dashed.

Low positive

These dread words seem designed to put women through an extra hell. A 'low positive' pregnancy test means that your pregnancy hormones haven't reached very high levels, and there's a 50/50 chance you're pregnant. This may be due to the embryo implanting very late, and it may go on to do so, or it can mean that implantation has failed and your period is about to start, or that there's an ectopic pregnancy. You will know within days – either because your period starts or because you have further tests which come out positive – which way your pregnancy is going. While you're enduring this further wait, it's easy to get despondent.

If you're pregnant, an ultrasound scan a couple of weeks later will confirm this. It also allows clinic staff to check that the pregnancy has implanted well in the uterus and to count the number of gestational sacs. You can expect several more scans in the early part of your pregnancy to check that everything's developing normally. If it is, you'll be referred back to your GP and you can make the transition to antenatal care – a journey we pick up again on p. 235.

Chances of success

One of the most important things to remember about IVF is that, statistically, it's much more likely not to work than it is to be successful – although a treatment which offers a 25 per cent chance of conception each cycle is comparable to the success rates for couples without any fertility problems for conceiving each month. All sorts of things can go wrong:

- sometimes the woman doesn't respond well to the drugs that control ovulation and the treatment cycle has to be cancelled before the eggs are collected
- sometimes only one or two eggs are retrieved, either because only that number developed or, despite the best will in the world, ovulation had already occurred by the time the collection was scheduled. Occasionally, no eggs are retrieved
- sometimes the eggs don't fertilise, so there are no embryos to transfer
- sometimes the embryos don't develop well enough to be implanted
- fairly often two or three good-quality embryos are transferred but implantation doesn't take place
- Although a pregnancy may result it may be miscarried

Although some couples do have their treatment cycles abandoned, the result for most couples – even those who have come all the way to embryo transfer with everything looking good – is a negative pregnancy test. After all that hope, stress, prayers and (for the majority), money, this 'failure' can be a crushing blow. Angela 'cried and cried' when she was told the news. She had several sessions with a counsellor before she felt strong enough, physically and emotionally, to go on to another cycle.

'I needed time to learn that what I was dealing with was not anger at the doctors, or nature, for everything having failed, and not disappointment in myself, or my husband either. Everyone involved had given it their all and been so caring. But the leftover feelings I had were those of grief – grief for the baby I was so sure would come this time.'

Unfortunately, the impression given by many TV programmes and magazine articles is that most couples will emerge from the process of IVF with their longed-for baby. Matt feels that,

'It's easy to get your hopes up too high and forget about the actual chances of it being successful, especially when you've tried everything else and this is the last resort – you feel it's bound to work.'

Sara also feels that

'You might hear of one IVF baby, but not the fifteen failed treatment cycles that went on at the same time.'

Anne found it hard to hang on to reality at her patient support group when she was undergoing IVF.

'People really do latch onto statistics. They bandy figures about: "This centre has a 25 per cent take-home-baby rate . . ." I thought, "What if we're in the other 75 per cent?" Let's face it, after all, we were all more likely to be.'

Research[5] shows that the most significant factors affecting the outcome of IVF treatment are:

- the age of the woman (the success rate steadily diminishes as she gets older)
- the quality of the sperm
- the duration of the infertility
- whether the woman has had a previous pregnancy
- how many IVF treatments the woman has had

For some couples, though, there is the joy of success. Alison underwent two cycles of AI, but on the third cycle her ovaries produced a large number of eggs and her consultant decided not to proceed because of the risk of a multiple pregnancy.

'They didn't want to waste the eggs, though, so they switched us to IVF, and that worked first time. We were delighted.'

Micromanipulation techniques

The term 'micromanipulation' refers to techniques used in IVF to bypass the zona pellucida, the protein shell which surrounds the egg:

- *intracytoplasmic sperm injection (ICSI)*: a relatively new technique which uses microinjection equipment to inject a single sperm directly through the zona pellucida into the centre of the egg
- *subzonal insemination (SUZI)*: a single sperm is placed just beneath the zona pellucida

Until a few years ago, the only option open to couples with severe male factor infertility was to try for a child using donor sperm. However, micromanipulation techniques (ICSI is the one most commonly used in the UK) have begun to offer a real alternative. Because only one sperm is required to be injected into the egg, ICSI and SUZI can be of great benefit to couples where the man has been diagnosed with a low sperm count, low numbers of motile sperm, poor forward progression of sperm, or a high proportion of sperm with abnormalities, all of which reduce the chances of fertilisation. These techniques can also be used to help men with a sperm blockage (where no sperm at all gets through to the semen) as sperm can be obtained from the epididymis (using MESA or PESA) or from the testicles (TESE) with a fine needle under anaesthetic.

————————————————ICSI————————————————

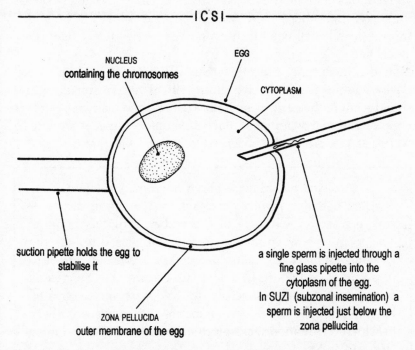

NUCLEUS
containing the chromosomes

EGG

CYTOPLASM

suction pipette holds the egg to
stabilise it

ZONA PELLUCIDA
outer membrane of the egg

a single sperm is injected through a
fine glass pipette into the
cytoplasm of the egg.
In SUZI (subzonal insemination) a
sperm is injected just below the
zona pellucida

In addition, couples who have had IVF cycles in which no fertilisation occurred, or in which there were very low rates of fertilisation, may find ICSI of benefit in overcoming their problems in egg/sperm interaction. Eggs will still need to be collected using the usual IVF methods.

The use of micromanipulation techniques is increasing, as is its success rate as measured in the live birth rate. Many clinics now find that their clinical pregnancy rates are as high as those achieved using conventional IVF methods.

However it is such a new technique, that assessment of the risks involved is only at an early stage. There is some concern that because ICSI involves piercing the egg it may cause a higher incidence of congenital abnormalities or problems with mental development. The results of studies vary – although most show that the risk from IVF/ICSI is no greater than when using conventional IVF alone. Because so few babies (relatively speaking) have been born worldwide as a result of IVF/ICSI, much more research will need to be done before significant figures are available.

In the meantime, reflecting these concerns, most clinics will advise couples who conceive through ICSI to have regular ultrasound scans in the early weeks of pregnancy, and many suggest that couples consider whether to have an amniocentesis at around 15 weeks. If you are at all concerned, ask your consultant.

'Assisted hatching': embryo micromanipulation

Assisted hatching involves creating an opening in the outer covering (zona pellucida) of the embryo after fertilisation. This form of embryo micromanipulation is used to help the growing embryo to emerge from its covering in order to implant in the uterus. The procedure has increased implantation rates, especially for older women. Assisted hatching can be used in conjunction with any procedure in which fertilisation takes place in the laboratory, including IVF and ICSI.

Pre-implantation genetic diagnosis

It's now possible to detect, before implantation, whether embryos created through IVF treatment carry genes which mean that the baby would be born with a serious inherited disorder such as cystic fibrosis or thalassemia. Only a few centres are currently licensed to carry out pre-implantation genetic diagnosis (PGD), and it's still at an early stage of development; but it's inevitable that, as we learn more about the genes responsible for such disorders, more and more people will want to avail themselves of the opportunities that this technique offers. In addition, it can be used to determine the sex of an embryo. In the UK, sex-selection of embryos is permitted only for couples who risk passing on a sex-linked disorder, like Duchenne's muscular dystrophy, which only affects male children. The man's sperm are sorted and injected into the eggs, and the sex of the resulting embryos is checked before they are replaced in the uterus. The HFEA is currently working with the Advisory Committee on Genetic Testing to produce guidance on the circumstances in which PGD would and would not be acceptable.

Cloning

From time to time, items in newspapers draw our attention to the prospect of cloning and its application to human fertility. One Italian embryologist has stated that he intends to create the first human clone with the aim of enabling infertile men to have children. Using techniques similar to those which produced Dolly the sheep, the world's first successful clone of an adult mammal, a cell would be taken from the man's body and the nucleus removed and treated. This treatment 'resets' the DNA of the nucleus so that a cell will behave as if it is a newly fertilised embryo. This nucleus would then be inserted into the woman's egg, from which the egg cell's own genetic material had been removed. The resulting embryo, if successfully implanted in her uterus, would grow into a clone of the man.

Leaving aside the technological barriers which would have to be conquered before the process was safe or routinely successful (it took 277 attempts to make Dolly), the idea of cloning a human being raises uncomfortable ethical questions. Although such a child would have the same DNA as his father, he would not be an exact physical or mental copy because of the environmental influences that affect the development of the individual. Nevertheless, the resemblances might be strong enough to cause psychological problems between father and son.

The European Parliament has attempted to outlaw human cloning but the decision still rests with individual countries. In the UK, while not technically illegal, the practice is blocked by the HFEA, which has declared that it will refuse a licence for such work. It is important to remember, therefore, that cloning is not yet a practical possibility in this country, and it is a technique that would benefit very few infertile couples anyway. Besides, most couples who want a child want exactly that, a unique individual child, not a copy of a living person.

GAMETE INTRAFALLOPIAN TRANSFER (GIFT)

GIFT is similar to IVF in that the woman's ovaries are stimulated and the eggs are collected, and the man also needs to produce sperm (or donor sperm can be used). The main difference between GIFT and IVF is that fertilisation occurs inside rather than outside the body. Once egg collection is complete, the eggs are assessed by an embryologist and up to three of the 'best' are mixed with around a hundred thousand motile sperm. The eggs and sperm are then immediately placed in the woman's fallopian tube in the same operation. GIFT is done either via a laparoscopy under general anaesthetic on a day-patient basis, or by using a catheter passed through the cervix, for which a local anaesthetic and sedation can be used. After that, the cycle proceeds as for IVF.

GIFT is often suggested to couples with unexplained infertility, where there might be problems with the cervical mucus, or where the woman has mild endometriosis. Obviously she will need to have at least one fallopian tube in working order, but GIFT is not recommended for women who have already had an ectopic pregnancy (and perhaps lost one fallopian tube) because of the risk of another.

While the success rates for GIFT are higher than those for IVF – partly, it seems because the developing embryos pass down the tube and into the uterus just as they would in a natural pregnancy – if it doesn't work it's harder to figure out why. Once the eggs and sperm are inside the woman's body, if no pregnancy results you can't tell whether fertilisation even took place. This is one reason why IVF may be recommended to some couples as a first option in order to establish the ability of the sperm to fertilise the eggs. If at least one fallopian tube is normal and fertilisation has occurred in vitro, GIFT may be appropriate if future treatment is needed.

As only three eggs can be transferred, any 'spare' ones will have to perish unless your clinic is licensed for freezing embryos. Then, if you wish, the spare eggs could be mixed with sperm and any resulting embryos could be frozen and stored for use in a future treatment cycle.

GIFT

Advantages

- it doesn't require a licence from the HFEA unless donor eggs or sperm are used, so you may find more centres near you offering this treatment
- it has a reasonably high success rate in comparison to IVF (in some centres as high as 30 per cent if the man's sperm count is within the normal range)
- embryo culture isn't required so in some clinics GIFT can be cheaper than IVF
- any resulting embryos will develop in the natural surroundings of the fallopian tube, not, as in IVF, in an artificial imitation of that environment
- it offers a good way forward for couples who are uncomfortable, for personal or religious reasons, with the idea of creating embryos outside the body

Disadvantages

- it can be invasive for a woman as surgery is usually required, with all the side-effects and physical repercussions of a general anaesthetic
- there seems to be an increased risk of twins or triplets
- if pregnancy does not result, it is hard to tell whether fertilisation was achieved or not. As with IVF, the ovaries need to be stimulated, and this can give rise to complications

ZYGOTE INTRAFALLOPIAN TRANSFER (ZIFT)

The term 'zygote' describes an egg just after fertilisation and before cell division has started. ZIFT is a mixture of IVF and GIFT; fertilisation occurs in the laboratory, just as it does with IVF. Three zygotes are then transferred to the woman's fallopian tube, much sooner than would be the case in IVF, because it is believed that the natural environment of the body is a better place to encourage an embryo to develop than a laboratory dish.

However, there are disadvantages to ZIFT, the main one being that the woman has to undergo two invasive procedures – egg collection and then laparoscopy – in quick succession. Also, some doctors feel that the opportunity to select the best three embryos to transfer is lost with ZIFT, because when the zygotes are transferred it is impossible to tell which are developing most promisingly.

FROZEN EMBRYOS

During IVF treatment, several embryos may be produced. As the law only allows up to three embryos to be transferred to a woman during any one treatment cycle, there may be some 'spare'. When embarking upon IVF, therefore, or if you are donating genetic material, you need to consider the future of any embryos created in this way.

If the clinic has the appropriate storage facilities, your 'spare' embryos can be frozen in liquid nitrogen for use in a further treatment cycle. Spare eggs from a GIFT cycle can also be fertilised in the laboratory and frozen in the same way. (This applies to the UK, but some countries ban or restrict the freezing of embryos; for example, in Germany they can only be frozen before the first cell division of the fertilised egg takes place.)

Freezing embryos means that you could avoid the need for repeating the processes of egg retrieval, sperm collection and fertilisation in any subsequent IVF cycle, making treatment much less stressful. If you decide that you don't want to freeze the remaining embryos, you could donate them for the treatment of other couples or for research, or you could allow them to perish. If you feel very strongly that you want to avoid having 'spare' embryos and facing these decisions, you may like to discuss with your doctor in advance the levels of drugs you are being given for superovulation to see if they are likely to result in a large number of eggs and therefore, possibly, embryos. As different women respond differently to these drugs, the exact numbers of developing follicles can never be ascertained, but you can make your feelings known. You could also request, if many eggs are produced, that not all of them are fertilised.

You will need to sign a consent form if you want to store your embryos, and the HFEA *Code of Practice* stresses the importance of counselling at this point so that couples can give informed consent. Some clinics force couples to consider such matters as who the embryos will belong to if the couple later divorce or separate, or what will happen to the embryos if one partner dies.

Jayne felt she had little choice about freezing her embryos:

'I'd hyperstimulated during the first part of the IVF cycle and produced 25 eggs, and the HRT injections to thicken my endometrium hadn't worked, so they decided they couldn't replace the embryos in that cycle, so we had to have them frozen.'

Many human embryos are now frozen: some authorities estimate that as many as half a million are in storage worldwide. Attitudes to these frozen embryos vary widely: some couples see them as no more than frozen genetic material, while others regard them as potential human life, and yet others as actual human life. Majella, who had one daughter following IVF treatment and also had three embryos frozen, admits that she thought of them as 'my triplets' while waiting to start another treatment cycle.

However, not all embryos make it through the thawing process, just as 'fresh' embryos don't always make it through the selection process or the implantation itself, and this is something Majella had to face.

'It was a very sad day, the day I went down to London and found that all of my triplets had gone.'

Anne and John also embarked upon IVF using their frozen embryos, but it wasn't a happy experience. Anne says,

'The first cycle I went through all the treatment to get me just right, and then they did a blood test and said they'd just missed the right point in the cycle so we had to abandon that attempt. So we had to start all over again and the next time they told us that the embryos had perished in the thawing process. That was hard, because not only do you get your body all ready, you also get your mind ready. And we knew IVF had worked for us before, so we had got our hopes it would work again.'

However, many thousands of babies all over the world have started life as frozen embryos and, although the success rate for IVF cycles is slightly lower for frozen embryos than for 'fresh' ones, the technique can help couples to create the family they hope for.

The statutory storage period for embryos is five years, although this can be extended to ten on request. Some women, including those undergoing chemotherapy or who have had a premature menopause, are allowed to store embryos until their 55th birthday. At the end of the storage period, embryos must be treated in one of the following ways, according to the couple's wishes:

- thawed for use in a further IVF cycle
- thawed and donated to others
- used for research
- allowed to perish

Not many people find such decisions easy, which is why counselling at the time of the original consent to freeze the embryos is so important. Nobody else can make these choices for you, but they can help you think them through. Even so, it may be several years after the original freezing that you are pushed into making a decision.

Alison and Peter had two embryos frozen after their first attempt at IVF had produced five. (Three had been replaced, and a son was born.) Out of the blue one day they received a letter asking them to decide what to do with these two embryos by a certain date. Alison says,

'All these dilemmas reduced to "Tick the box" without any opportunity for further discussion. It was strange.'

It is hardly surprising that some couples find it hard to decide the fate of their frozen embryos. Sometimes finance comes into decisions: Ilona says,

'We've got two frozen embryos still stored at the clinic where we had our IVF treatment, but we're not eligible for any more NHS treatment and we can't afford private treatment, so we won't be able to use them unless we win the Lottery. It seems very sad to think that we can't follow this through because of lack of money, but I think we have to face the fact that one day they'll be destroyed.'

If you have had embryos frozen and then decide not to use them, you can leave them in the hands of the hospital to perish or you may want to ask to take them home and bury them. Only you know how important these small cells, no bigger than a full stop, are to you. If you do feel they carry the potential for human life, you may want to acknowledge the bereavement you feel when that life will never happen.

DO WE DO IT AGAIN?

Whatever means of assisted conception you've used, if your treatment has resulted in 'failure' especially if it's your first time, you will want to try again as soon as you can. Sometimes there are physical barriers. Eilish found that the fertility drugs she took caused cysts in her ovaries.

'They were just "left-over" follicles that didn't shrink after ovulation. Some got quite big but they disappeared quickly, so I only had to wait one cycle for them to disappear and then I could try again. Not all women get them, I know. I'm just susceptible. Like I'm not susceptible to getting pregnant.'

Whether you can try again depends on whether your health authority will fund you for further treatment or, if you are paying for your own treatment, whether you can afford it. Gail is currently trying to weigh up the choices after the failure of her second IUI:

'I'm going to see the consultant next week and I hope to move on to IVF next cycle. I did get pregnant naturally two years ago so there's a good chance that another IUI will work, but I have mild endo and that may have got worse. We could have a laparoscopy to check, but that's a few hundred pounds in itself, and if it did show something was wrong, we'd have to move to IVF anyway.'

Some couples will be limited to a maximum of three cycles of IVF treatment through funding from their health authority. Even couples who have the resources, both financial and emotional, to consider more do wonder when enough is enough. Do you stop after three cycles? Four? Five? Ten? It's not an easy decision to make. Some couples will achieve pregnancy on their second or third attempt, although statistics suggest that success rates go down from the fourth cycle onwards. However, this could simply be because the women attempting a fourth cycle are older, or the causes of their infertility are more complex.

Sara underwent several cycles of IVF and her consultant tried to persuade her to stop:

'She kept saying "It won't work for you, you just have to accept that," but we weren't ready to accept it. We had set ourselves a limit, but it wasn't her limit. I remember sitting in her office with my tears dripping on the table, pleading, "Just one more go, just one more go." So the consultant said to us, "This is your last attempt," and, of course, it wasn't a good attempt. We only got two embryos, and we didn't expect it to work, so we were quite despondent. But the next morning the embryologist phoned us up and said that, even though there were only two embryos, they were of really good quality. He said, "If I had twenty embryos, I'd only put these two back." And it worked. Even though our consultant wasn't optimistic, even though it was our last go, it worked. We actually had a twin implantation and then we got Thomas. It took us 14 years to have him, and I'm just so glad we went that bit further.'

Not everyone is as lucky as Sara, and the decision about when to stop can be difficult for all concerned. There is more about the feelings involved in stopping treatment in Chapter 12.

6

Donation

For some couples, straightforward assisted conception treatments are not enough. Sometimes, perhaps because of early menopause or an inherited condition such as Turner's syndrome, a woman may not be able to produce any eggs, or she may have received surgery or chemotherapy which has left her sterile. In such situations, IVF using donated eggs fertilised by her partner's sperm will be needed if the couple are to achieve pregnancy. In other cases, the woman may be a carrier of an inheritable disease such as Duchenne's muscular dystrophy or haemophilia, and the couple are unwilling to risk giving birth to a child who may suffer greatly and die at an early age. While techniques are being developed to identify which embryos might be affected, such tests are not readily available and the couple may request egg donation instead, feeling that it offers them a greater chance of having a healthy child.

Using donated eggs is also a choice taken up by many older women. Women in their forties have a very low chance of success conceiving with IVF using their own eggs. If a woman has been having treatments for many years and now feels that time is running out, the couple may decide that using a younger woman's eggs offers them their only chance to have a child.

Donation can help in cases of male infertility, too. A man may simply produce no sperm of his own, in which case the couple may find that donor insemination (DI) offers them their only chance of conceiving. DI can also help couples in which the man is carrying a genetic disorder which he doesn't want to pass on to any children. Insemination using donor semen is a tried-and-tested method of treatment and has been practised in the UK for many years. In this country alone, several thousand children have been born following DI and there are approximately 1500 such births each year. DI is also sometimes suggested for couples in which, although the man is producing sperm, those sperm are unable to fertilise the egg, and for couples where immune factors prevent fertilisation taking place. It can also help men who are unable to ejaculate because of neurological disorders. Although new techniques such as ICSI (intracytoplasmic sperm injection) now offer men the chance to become fathers using their own sperm in these instances, for many couples DI proves a better choice.

Donation and the law

Egg and sperm donations are regulated by the Human Fertilisation and Embryology Act, 1990. Amongst its provisions are:

- the donor will be anonymous: his or her name will be known only to the clinic and the HFEA
- while the HFEA may collect some information about donors (such as hair colour, eye colour, occupation and interests) this information may not be given to any child born as a result of the donation
- any payment for donors is restricted to £15 plus reasonable expenses
- the woman receiving the treatment and her husband or male partner will be the legal parents of any child

---

Except where donation is intentionally between people known to each other, all donations in the UK are regulated by the Human Fertilisation and Embryology Authority (HFEA) and anonymous. If someone donates sperm or eggs to help you while you are having fertility treatment, neither you nor any child born following the donation will ever know who the donor was. The donor will be the 'genetic parent' of any child born as a result of gamete donation, but not the 'legal parent'. You and your partner will be the legal parents of any child resulting from treatment using donated gametes. Donors have no legal relationship with, or any continuing responsibility to, any children born from the donation.

WHAT DOES BEING A DONOR INVOLVE?

While donation is a simple procedure for a man, he needs to be aware that his donation could result in the birth of up to ten children (in rare cases more, if a family request a sibling for a child already born from that donor's sperm). This limit has been imposed in order to reduce the chances of children growing up and marrying someone who is, unknown to them, genetically related: their half-brother or half-sister.

The children will not be able to trace their biological father. While men can donate sperm up to the age of 55, the HFEA is monitoring published evidence on whether the incidence of birth defects increases with paternal age. Sperm may be frozen and stored for up to ten years.

Egg donation is a more complex process. Egg donors need to be under 35 and preferably of proven fertility. The donor needs to receive a 10-day course of fertility drugs to stimulate her ovaries to produce several eggs. In addition, she needs to make at least an initial visit to the hospital or IVF centre for counselling and tests, a second visit for an ultrasound scan to see if the eggs are ripening, and a third visit for their removal. The eggs are collected in a surgical operation which lasts around 30 minutes. They are then either fertilised outside the body (IVF) and transferred to the womb of the recipient, or mixed with sperm and transferred into the fallopian tubes of the recipient (GIFT).

Donors must give written consent to the use and storage of their sperm or eggs, and of any embryos produced with them. Donors can consent to donate to treat others, or for a research project, for example. The law states that this must be 'informed consent', so all donors must be given information about the process and implications of donation, including any storage time, and they must have been offered counselling.

SCREENING

Clinics select all donors carefully. They must be of reasonable intelligence, fit and in good health. All are required to provide a full medical history before donating sperm or eggs, including details of any family history of hereditary disease. Donors are always advised to be open and honest so as to avoid future problems. (A situation in which a child born with an inherited disability, undisclosed by the donor, were to sue that donor for damages would be devastating.)

Many clinics screen donors for a wide range of diseases. This screening includes blood tests for hepatitis B and C, gonorrhoea and syphilis, and most will also perform a chromosome analysis to check for abnormalities.

Donors are also tested for the presence of HIV antibodies in their blood. The first test takes place before they are accepted, the second about six months later. This is because it can take several months for the presence of HIV antibodies to reach detectable proportions. During this 'HIV window', any donated material – sperm or embryos – is frozen. Currently eggs cannot be frozen due to the risk of damage, although research into 'oocyte cryopreservation' continues. Recipients, too, will be tested for HIV antibodies and hepatitis B and C.

Screening gamete donors for cystic fibrosis (CF) has become standard practice at most licensed clinics and is strongly recommended by the HFEA. (CF is an inherited disease which results in severe lung infections and breathing difficulties. Most people with CF die before they reach 21.) Clinics are required to inform couples receiving donated genetic material whether the donor has been tested for CF. Nevertheless, the test used to detect whether a person is a carrier of the gene that causes CF isn't infallible, since it only identifies approximately 85 per cent of carriers. Even if all donors are screened, therefore, there remains a small risk that a donor may be a CF carrier, and clinics must tell couples of these risks.

Donors must receive counselling before having these tests. Anyone agreeing to be tested for CF should be offered genetic counselling, as they will need information about what it implies for themselves and their families if it turns out that they are carriers.

You may wish to ask your clinic about their policy on screening egg and sperm donors.

How do they match a recipient to a donor?
Clinics record details of a donor's physical appearance – such as hair, skin and eye colour, as well as height, build and blood group – and then usually try to match these physical characteristics with those of the male or female partner whose eggs or sperm are to be replaced. An exact match, however, may be impossible to provide. If you are considering using donor eggs or sperm, you may wish to ask about the criteria your clinic uses when matching donors with couples.

CONSIDERING DONOR GAMETES

If you want to have DI or IVF using donor eggs, you must be offered counselling. While you may or may not want to take up this opportunity, there are some aspects which couples will want to think about and talk about between themselves before moving forward:

- are we both equally committed to this decision?
- is the partner who will not have a child who is their biological offspring still grieving the 'loss' of this child?
- does the father fear he may not feel close to a child born through DI?
- does the mother fear she may not feel close to a child born through egg donation?
- are they concerned that the child will not look like them?
- are they concerned that relatives will make comments about the child's difference?
- will they tell anyone about the donation? Are both partners in agreement on this?

It is important, if either partner has doubts about moving forward, that you take time to explore these before beginning treatment, and certainly before any child is born.

DONOR INSEMINATION

Penny recalls,

'When we found out that Donald wasn't producing any sperm at all, we had two choices. Either we could put ourselves on the list of couples waiting to adopt, or we could consider DI. We knew that the chances of being able to adopt were small, and any child conceived as a result of the DI would be biologically closer to us because he would share some genetic traits with me. It also meant I was able to experience pregnancy, giving birth and breastfeeding. . . . In fact, as soon as we found out I was pregnant, then the pregnancy continued just the way any other would.'

Sperm donation is a long-established procedure, and some reports estimate that up to one in eight infertile couples are treated in this way. But obviously it isn't an answer for couples in which the woman also has fertility problems. Around 50 per cent of couples will achieve a pregnancy following treatment with donor sperm; the number of treatment cycles required varies, but six is an average. All the semen used in DI is frozen and thawed just before use. There is no evidence that freezing affects the sperm, and couples using DI don't run any increased risk of producing a baby with developmental or chromosomal abnormalities.

If a couple decide to have DI, the man will be asked to sign a consent form agreeing to the treatment. He will then become the legal father of any child conceived as a result, and his name will appear on the birth certificate.

The way DI treatments are carried out varies between clinics. Some recommend the use of drugs with DI to ensure that the woman is ovulating, while others prefer to rely on the woman using ovulation predictor kits. The number of inseminations done in each cycle can also vary, as can the method used – the sperm can be put into the vagina, the cervix or the uterus. (There is more information about insemination on p. 111.) Ask about these things at your clinic before beginning treatment. Also, find out how many cycles they generally offer: some have a limit.

Male fertility is astonishingly unpredictable. Men with extremely low sperm counts have gone on to father children. Men with extremely high sperm counts sometimes seem unable to have a child. This is one reason why the decision to opt for donor insemination can be so fraught for a couple. Unless there is a definite reason why the man cannot have a child – for example, he is producing no sperm at all – it can be a difficult decision to make. You may also find that your doctor is unwilling to recommend DI as a suitable way forward if he feels there are alternatives.

Kate and Mike's only hope of having children lay in donor insemination, but even so they had reservations. Says Kate,

'The decision to have DI was complex. We both saw it as a positive alternative, but I was assailed by religious and moral scruples. I was also filled with revulsion at the depersonalised means of conception and the facelessness of the donor. Painfully, we worked through these

*conflicting reactions before committing ourselves to DI. We were open
about it with our family and friends and invested all our hopes in it. I
was inseminated on two or three days each cycle. It was hugely
draining: arranging time off work, travelling to the hospital and, above
all, surviving the emotional peaks and troughs. Our lives were on hold:
we were consumed by the struggle for a baby and became socially
isolated. After about a year, the need for a less fraught existence began
to overtake the longing for a pregnancy. I went through about 16 cycles
before we decided to stop.'*

As Kate makes clear, the use of sperm from another man to help a
couple conceive a child they desperately want is not something
undertaken lightly. There are moral, philosophical, and possibly
religious aspects which each couple needs to consider, think
through and accept. This is one reason why the HFEA insists on
counselling for couples contemplating DI.

All donations in the UK (except under special circumstances,
when a clinic agrees to a couple using the sperm of someone known
to them, such as the man's brother) must be anonymous. Nevertheless, there has been some speculation recently that couples with
definite ideas of what they do and don't want their donor to look
like, or who have the desire to include particular traits in their
child's potential make-up, will make connections with American
sperm banks. There they can find out information about a variety of
potential donors, and many banks will send photographs. After
making your choice and a credit card payment, sperm could be
delivered to your door by courier . . . This is not an impossible
scenario, even though the HFEA would insist that you have a
licence to import the sperm and would want to check that it had
been screened properly.

Penny, whose son Robert was conceived through DI, can see
why such an idea might be attractive:

*'I do wonder sometimes about the biological father. I know the story
that most sperm donors are medical students, and I know they've all*

been through a rigorous screening process so I'm not worried about that aspect. But just now and again, I see something in Robert and I wonder. Is that from me? Or from someone we'll never know?'

Some couples who have DI are advised to continue having intercourse during the cycle in which insemination is carried out, so the possibility exists that the child might be biologically theirs alone. Penny is not so sure that this is a good idea:

'I think it introduces one more uncertainty into a situation that's already uncertain. I think if you're doing that, then DI is probably not for you anyway. For us, we had to reach a point where the genetic contribution didn't matter. What mattered was the child we were going to have together.'

WHERE DO EGG DONORS COME FROM?

No payments (apart from travel expenses) can be made to a woman for donating eggs, so all egg donors do so voluntarily. Often donors are relatives or friends of a woman who needs donated eggs; others have responded to recent media campaigns highlighting the shortage of egg donors. Some women who are undergoing sterilisation themselves offer to donate eggs at the same time. Sometimes women undergoing IVF treatment produce more eggs than they can use in their own treatment cycle, and choose to donate these to others.

Frances remembers how she first came to consider donating eggs:

'My children have given me infinite pleasure: the moment when the little stick turned blue was the happiest of my life. If I hadn't been able to get pregnant, I don't know how I would have coped. I became friends with another expectant mother in my first antenatal class. Her baby girl was born with a genetically transmitted syndrome which caused her to die before her first birthday. A second girl was born with the same syndrome and died at four months. I offered my eggs, but my friend's

husband couldn't cope with this. Luckily, she went on to have a healthy baby boy. But I began to think that, if I could consider donating for a friend, I could donate anonymously to help another woman. As a postnatal supporter for the National Childbirth Trust, I began to meet women who had problems getting pregnant. The idea of becoming an egg donor stayed with me, so I could help someone have the joy I had in my own children. My partner was happy for me to become an egg donor but wanted to wait until we had completed our family. He was concerned that some part of the process might affect my own fertility. I was fairly sure there was no risk, but wanted to respect his feelings. After our third baby, we decided to investigate donation.'

Women donating eggs need to go through all the stresses and face all the risks that accompany ovarian stimulation and egg collection. Frances, however, didn't find the process too disruptive to the rest of her life:

'The clinic opens at 7 a.m., so I could dash in, have an injection and a blood test and be home in time to walk my oldest child to school. The clinic staff had hoped that I would produce about twelve follicles with an egg in each, and two recipients would be able to get six. However, I only produced eight, so one recipient was given them all. There was no reason for this – women respond in different ways to the process. My eggs were collected using the ultrasound-guided needle, but I had a general anaesthetic as I wanted to feel nothing. I was sent to sleep and woke up back on the ward. My stomach ached, but no more than with a bad period. I had some painkillers and was soon feeling fine.'

Nevertheless, perhaps because women who want to donate eggs have to dose their bodies with hormones and undergo surgery (quite unlike the procedure associated with sperm donation) there is a national shortage of egg donors. All the clinics offering this treatment in the UK have couples on their waiting lists. As a result, getting treatment when you need egg donation is not always easy, as Sara found:

'I phoned every centre in the country about egg donation to see if they would treat us. Some lists were completely closed. Others didn't want to put us on their lists because we'd have to wait so long for treatment.'

For a couple who need egg donation, this extra wait is doubly frustrating as the need for donation may only become apparent after years of unsuccessful infertility treatment – to face a further long wait (between two and five years is normal) can be a devastating blow. The needs of women from a variety of ethnic cultures are also not being met. Most egg donors are white, so the waiting lists for women of other cultures are even longer. Sara says,

'I've met 17-year-olds who have gone through an early menopause and their only chance of having children will be through egg donation, and they're told "Put yourself on the waiting list now." They're not even in a steady relationship, they're not even thinking about having children yet, but they need to go on the waiting list so that if they ever do want children, they have a chance of being near the top.'

The recent campaigns to increase awareness of the need for egg donors were designed to alleviate such problems. One debate has been about whether payment to egg donors would help ease this situation. Egg donors are paid in other countries, but in the UK there is a tradition of donating for medical reasons (such as giving blood) through altruism and not for profit. A legal loophole that allowed women to sell their eggs through an agency raised fears that the whole enterprise might become commercialised. Mary Sidebotham, (the Donor Recruitment Co-ordinator for the National Gamete Donation Society) is against payment.

'Real expenses should be paid so a woman is not out of pocket, but how do you put a price on life? I think it is easier to give away something of yourself than to sell it. And this is a gift of love. If a donor is focusing on the money, it means they're blocking their minds off from what they're

doing. They're doing it for all the wrong reasons. A woman has to be sure she isn't going to be looking into prams in years to come.'

Krystyna, however, who became pregnant through egg donation while living in the United States, has experienced the benefits of the American approach. She was treated at the Bay Area Clinic in California, where she and her husband were living following his temporary job relocation there.

'We felt fortunate to have been in America. In Britain, we would have been considered too old for treatment. Also, the ban on the sale of eggs which means donors can't be paid has resulted in an extreme shortage of donors. We paid our donor a £1500 fee as well as all her medical expenses following the American Infertility Society's guidelines for compensation for risk and time involved.'

Krystyna did not need to wait for treatment, and was happy in herself as to the motives of her donor:

'Since donors are paid a fee in America, they are screened to ensure their motives are altruistic. We were given copies of their completed questionnaires which showed us their physical characteristics, educational background, hobbies and interests, as well as answers to such questions as "Why do you want to become a donor?" and "What message would you give to the recipient of your eggs?" All donors were screened medically, genetically and psychologically for diseases, inherited conditions like Tay-Sachs, sickle-cell anaemia and haemophilia, family history and their commitment to the donor process.'

Yet in this country, even setting aside the issue of whether payment would ease the situation, there are pressures. In many treatment centres, couples are told that if they can recruit an egg donor they will go to the top of the waiting list. They won't receive the eggs of the donor they introduce to the clinic, as the law requires all donations to be anonymous, but this admission to the 'fast track' does place an added burden on some couples at an already difficult time. Sara and David put all their efforts into this:

'We must have spent thousands on adverts and writing articles to spark interest in our plight, trying to recruit someone who would donate eggs so that we could go to the top of the list.'

More and more couples are trying to obtain egg donors via the Internet, publicising details of their situation and giving the address of the hospital at which they are being treated so that potential donors can get in touch. The desperation of many couples is all too apparent.

CHOOSING EGG DONATION

Krystyna says,

'Egg donation was something we initially dismissed. It seemed to belong to the realms of science fiction: something out of Brave New World *and not for us. There were three main reasons why we changed our minds. Firstly, we were attracted by the much higher success rates it would offer us. I had climbed the ladder of escalating infertility treatments, starting with ovulation kits – squinting at coloured dots trying to convince myself – then months of intrauterine inseminations, and our infertility treatments had culminated in two failed IVF cycles which didn't even reach the retrieval or embryo-transfer stage as I never produced enough eggs. Egg donation offered us the best chance of getting pregnant. Secondly, the risks of Down's syndrome and other chromosomal birth defects, which were frighteningly high at my age, 42, would be much lower. It's the age of the eggs, not the uterus, which is significant. Our donor was 27. Finally, we liked it better than the alternatives of surrogacy or adoption. I would have the opportunity to experience pregnancy and childbirth, and to breastfeed my baby.'*

Deciding that you will try to conceive with donated eggs can sometimes be difficult, as Sara found:

'Nobody had ever been able to give us a definite reason why we couldn't have a child using my own eggs – that was the thing. They thought there must be some environmental or chromosomal damage, but they weren't sure. When you know it's the only way, perhaps if you've gone through a premature menopause, then I think it must be easier because the decision is taken out of your hands. I initially felt pressured into going through with it because I hadn't really come to terms with accepting it wasn't going to work with my own eggs, that I wasn't going to have a baby with my own genetic material. In fact, I couldn't go through with the first treatment. I pulled out when the donor was just starting stimulants. I told the Programme Co-ordinator that I was having problems and she directed me to a counsellor who said we had to stop this now.'

Sara was glad she stopped, as she needed time to come to terms with what was happening. David, her partner, tried to reassure her, saying,

'It's just an egg. You're the one who's going to give it life.'

But it took Sara a while to accept that. Gradually she talked through her fears and feelings with a counsellor until she got to the heart of her doubts:

'Specifically, I didn't feel that the baby would be mine. I was worried about seeing a stranger come out of me, as if I was going to give birth to some alien.'

There were others factors at work, too.

'It wasn't just the worries about the donated eggs. The grief from our previous miscarriages was so overwhelming, and I knew that there was

a very low chance of us being successful, so I was partly reluctant to face that grief again.'

Krystyna feels that

'It is inevitable that there will be some grieving for the loss of your genetic child who will never be born, but I was only too happy to be pregnant to grieve for very long.'

A BABY FROM DONATED EGGS

The process of assisted conception using donated eggs has to be precisely timed and coordinated. On the day when the eggs are collected from the donor, the man needs to provide a semen sample, so that the eggs can be mixed with the sperm and – it is hoped – fertilisation will take place.

At the same time, the recipient's body must itself be hormonally prepared for pregnancy. Her own ovulation cycle is suppressed and the endometrium thickened so that it's ready for implantation of the embryos. This means further medication, along with ultrasound scans to check that the endometrium is growing as it should. Sara found this part of the process hard work:

'They start the recipient off very early, so I was thrown into the menopause for two or three months at a time just so I could be ready when the donor came through. It was gruelling, but a small price to pay.'

When all the conditions are right, the embryos will be placed in the recipient's uterus through her vagina and cervix using a fine catheter. This may be uncomfortable – rather like having a cervical smear test. She will need to take progesterone supplements at least until a pregnancy test can be done (about 14 days later) and, if she is pregnant, these will continue for several more weeks.

Even if everything goes well physically and hormonally, a treatment cycle involving egg donation is probably harder to deal with than a straight IVF cycle because of the complex emotions involved on all sides. Sara says,

'I found IVF with donated eggs much harder than having IVF with my own eggs. First there was all this waiting, all this uncertainty, and knowing that this person could pull out at any moment . . . At our second attempt, I'd gone through protracted treatment to get me ready to receive the eggs and then our donor changed her mind. And we had to share her with someone else. I know that sounds strange, but egg donors are in such short supply that sometimes there are three recipients waiting for one person's eggs. It's the waiting that's definitely the hardest.'

Krystyna's experience was different, partly because she was able to choose her donor:

'We chose our donor from a book with pictures of women (some of them glamour shots!) from the clinic's donor bank, the largest in northern California. It felt a little like choosing a baby out of a catalogue. When selecting a donor, it was tempting to try to improve on the original: here was my chance to pick a blonde with blue eyes. In the end, we chose the woman who most resembled me physically so that our baby might be genetically believable, even though some genetic families aren't believable, either.'

Krystyna was also given another option:

'We were given the choice of anonymous, semi-anonymous or open relationship with the donor, and decided on partial anonymity. We didn't get to meet her, but I did write to thank her and let her know I'd got pregnant with her eggs. I've also kept a photo of her and her daughter which she had specially taken for me so that I would have something to remember her by.'

For Sara:

*'We wanted to stay anonymous. I wouldn't have wanted to meet her.
I'd had a "profile" of her, so knew she had brown hair and brown eyes
like I did, and she was a psychology graduate – as I am – so there was
an affinity there, too, but I didn't want to know any more than that. I
didn't want to see her. I was frightened that I'd then look at the baby
and actually see her. I thought that knowing about us might be difficult
for her, as well. I didn't want her to worry about us and what was
happening in our lives.'*

Even in situations where donors and recipients don't meet, women
receiving the donated eggs have a sense of connection with their
donor and an appreciation of what she is doing for them. Sara says,

*'On the day she was having her egg collection, I took flowers and a card
to the IVF unit and asked the staff to pass them on to my donor when
she came round from the operation.'*

Krystyna also remembers that

*'Throughout the treatment, I worried about bumping into my donor in
hospital corridors. I imagined every woman sitting in the infertility
clinic was her, and I fantasised about meeting her. I felt some guilt
about what we were putting her through and the impact of treatment
upon her. But, above all, the overwhelming feeling I had for her was
complete and utter awe. I marvelled at how someone could have done
this for us. Becoming a donor takes a rare kind of individual. Not
everyone can go through what a donor goes through, all for a child that
can never be hers.'*

Most donors in the UK are curious to know if their efforts have
achieved a pregnancy and some clinics will tell donors this, if they
want to ask. However, donors will be given no information about
the outcome of the pregnancy or any children born.

Krystyna's treatment was straightforward from her point of view. From the twelve eggs retrieved from the donor, six were fertilised and she and her husband obtained five viable pre-embryos. Here she was given another choice not open to women in the UK:

'We were able to choose how many to transfer and decided on all five. I felt that if the treatment didn't succeed, I'd always be thinking, "If only I had transferred that fifth one." The transfer itself was painless and took less than a minute. I then had three days' required bed rest. The ten days waiting for the results were agonising. We never expected egg donation to succeed at the first attempt. It was another three weeks before we found out that only one of the embryos had implanted. We'd been told that the risk of a multiple birth was about 50 per cent. There followed three months of ultrasound examinations to monitor the pregnancy and progesterone injections administered every evening by my husband – with a two-inch needle into my backside which eventually came to resemble a pincushion. I had an uncomplicated pregnancy and gave birth to a daughter.'

Nevertheless, if you are pregnant after having received donated eggs, you will receive careful monitoring. Some studies have shown that women who have become pregnant with donated eggs have a higher than usual risk of developing hypertension during pregnancy, of requiring a caesarean delivery and of having a post-partum haemorrhage.[6]

Sara, whose son Thomas was delivered early after she developed pre-eclampsia, also had a post-partum haemorrhage ('Everything, really') but still came through these trials with her joy undimmed:

'I cannot express our gratitude to our egg donor for making this possible for us.'

Krystyna thinks of her egg donor as

'a very warm and wonderful person who, through her courage and generosity, helped make our dream come true. Some couples are eager to dismiss their donor as soon as they become pregnant, but I'm proud of her and don't want to forget her.'

Frances, talking from a donor's viewpoint, also feels what she did was worthwhile:

'I'm very glad I donated eggs. Someone, somewhere will look down on her new baby, a baby she might have been told she could never have, and what can be more rewarding than that?'

Once the baby arrives, of course, he or she will inevitably be subjected to special scrutiny by parents and others. Sara says,

'Thomas doesn't look like either of us. He's got the greyest eyes. . . and very long fingers. . . . We said to each other at one point, "Do you think they put the right embryo back?" But when the photographer came to take his picture in the hospital, he said to me, "Oh, he's so like you." We just smiled and said we couldn't see it ourselves.'

Krystyna, too, has found:

'Since Andrea was born, I do get the inevitable comparisons in appearance: "She looks just like you," or, "She doesn't look a bit like you." "She has your eyes." "She has your nose." I quietly nod in agreement. Most of the time I have to remind myself that I'm not her genetic mother, but in the back of my mind I am always aware of our donor.'

TELLING THE CHILD

For parents with a child conceived by DI or through egg donation, a major issue is whether or not to tell that child about their origins. Unless you tell your child, he or she may never know.

The HFEA keeps a register of information about donors and the children born from donor treatments. While the identity of all donors is kept confidential, they are asked for their names and date of birth so that any future children can be told whether they are genetically related to someone they want to marry. The HFEA has a legal duty to tell all adults (aged 16 and over) who ask whether they were born as a result of treatment using donated eggs or sperm. However, the law states that the name of the donor cannot be given to someone who enquires in this way.

Richard, whose son was born as a result of DI, feels he ought to tell him that his genetic material came from someone else but doesn't feel he knows the right way to go about it.

'I mean, most couples don't tell their children all the details of their conception, do they? You might give a very general answer to the question "Where do babies come from?" but most couples wouldn't go into intricate detail about what happened on their honeymoon.'

Krystyna, however, feels that

'It is a child's irrevocable right to know about her origins and the circumstances of her birth. Honesty and openness are an inherent part of responsible parenthood.'

She has already begun telling her daughter.

'Rather than a one-time event – a single moment when the truth is "discovered" – I believe that telling should be a continuing, evolving process over the years. Since Andrea turned three, I have started to introduce the idea of "the donor lady who helped Mummy and Daddy to have you". My daughter sometimes asks, "How did she do that?" and I explain, "She did a wonderful thing and gave Mummy some of her eggs because Mummy's weren't working properly." Once, when I'd stopped in the High Street to chat to a woman I'd met at playgroup,

Andrea asked afterwards, "Is that her? The donor lady?" We've started making Andrea her own "My Family" book with pictures of her relatives and of her donor. As she grows and asks more questions, I will explain different aspects and give her more information. We also have a book I bought in America called Mummy, Did I Grow in Your Tummy?, which explains in a picture-story form all about the alternative ways of conceiving.'

While the law in the UK states at present that no information at all about the donor can be given to any future child, this may change. Donors are therefore asked to give in their own words some non-identifying information about themselves to the HFEA – for example, what they look like, what their talents and interests are – in case a child born as the result of the donation would find it helpful to know more about his or her genetic origins.

Frances explains her feelings about any children who might have been born as a result of her donation.

'I am aware that another woman is their mother in a way that I am not. I gave some genetic material – no more than that. If a baby born as a result of my donation contracted a disease such as a bone-marrow problem, I might be approached to give bone marrow, for example. I know it is highly unlikely, but I would be happy to help.'

Donors and recipients concur. The last word goes to Krystyna:

'I believe that society tends to overemphasise the importance of genes. The quality of parenting and the creation of a sense of family through a loving and caring relationship with the child is more important than biological parenthood. Now that Andrea is five and the bond between us grows deeper every day, if I was given the choice of living my life over again and having a child who was genetically mine or having our daughter the way we did, I would choose her every time. I don't believe I could love another child, even a biological one, as much as I love her. Even my husband, who was always a little ambivalent *about children, now feels "she's the best thing we've done". I don't share a single gene with my daughter but I do share much more – the magic of life and the miracle of raising her. Thanks to the woman who became my donor.'*

7

Surrogacy

S urrogacy is not a new invention – it has a long and distin-
guished pedigree. In the Old Testament it is recorded that
Sarah, Abraham's wife, enlisted her slave Hagar to carry a
child for her when she could not conceive herself. Thousands of
years ago Abraham had to have intercourse with Hagar, but
modern developments in artificial insemination techniques have
opened up the idea to couples for whom the idea of surrogacy
would otherwise have been repugnant. Despite all the recent
medical advances in the treatment of infertility, there will always
be couples who, for various reasons, cannot have a child of their
own. Sometimes the woman is unable to carry a child herself
because of abnormalities in her uterus, for example, or if she has
had a hysterectomy. In these instances, the only way the couple will
be able to have a child who is their genetic offspring is to enlist the
help of a woman who will carry and give birth to a child for them.
Nowadays, the success of IVF has meant that it is possible for a
couple to have their own eggs and sperm mixed in a laboratory and
implanted in another woman's womb, so that any resulting child is
genetically entirely their own.

Despite its history, surrogacy has never been without contro-
versy. Even Sarah and Hagar had arguments. There have been a few
extreme and well-publicised cases where the surrogate mother has
refused to hand over the baby to the intended parents. The
combination of money, lawyers and babies is a volatile mix.

Yet the vast majority of successful surrogate births don't receive any publicity. Kim Cotton, who herself achieved fame as Britain's first commercially paid surrogate mother, estimates that approximately 97 per cent of arrangements involving the support organisation she helped to set up, COTS, have reached happy conclusions. COTS has now been involved in over two hundred successful surrogate births, each of which has brought joy to a couple who couldn't otherwise have had children, and, not forgetting the other side of the equation, joy to the surrogates too.

Sometimes the surrogate is a sister or close friend of the infertile couple. More often she is a stranger, and arrangements are made with the help of a third party. In either case, surrogacy involves a huge amount of physical, emotional and financial commitment over an extended period of time, and should never be entered into without thorough consideration. You need to think through all the medical, legal, financial and emotional aspects before you start, not after. Although the rewards can be breathtaking when everything goes well, the consequences can be heartbreaking when they do not.

Why not adopt?

Adoption is, for many couples, a deeply satisfying alternative to a life without children. However, the social changes that have taken place over the last generation – more freely available contraception and abortion, shifting social attitudes to 'unmarried mothers' – have meant that the number of children being put forward for adoption has dropped significantly. There are more couples applying to adopt babies than there are babies who need to be adopted. For many couples, therefore, surrogacy is their only chance of becoming parents. In addition, surrogacy allows a couple to be closely involved with the pregnancy and birth in a way that adoption usually doesn't.

DIFFERENT TYPES OF SURROGACY

There are two types of surrogacy:

- *traditional (straight) surrogacy*, where the surrogate mother is also the biological mother. She is inseminated with the intended father's sperm at the appropriate point in her cycle and, if she conceives, carries the pregnancy to term. Any resulting child will have half the surrogate's genetic material from her own egg
- *gestational (host) surrogacy*, where both the egg and sperm of the intended parents are mixed using IVF techniques. The resulting embryos are placed into the surrogate (who may also have been given hormones to help time her cycle so that her body is ready for an embryo to implant). A gestational surrogate mother (sometimes called a 'carrier') has no genetic link to the child she carries

For Nichole, this difference was crucial when she was considering carrying a baby for another couple:

'I knew that the baby or babies would not be mine genetically or biologically, because they were made from the couple's eggs and sperm. I could not be inseminated. For me, that would be like giving away my own child because it was my own egg.'

The type of surrogacy arrangement that a couple will need depends on their particular difficulty with conceiving. A couple might consider traditional surrogacy if the woman cannot produce any eggs of her own. This may be because she has gone through an early menopause, has had chemotherapy which has destroyed her ovaries, or has severe endometriosis which has damaged her ovaries.

If a woman can produce her own eggs but cannot carry a baby, a couple might consider gestational surrogacy. If she has had a hysterectomy, for example, or has a severe congenital abnormality of the uterus, she could never become pregnant. In addition, some women have heart or kidney disease, severe diabetes or illnesses which need management by drugs potentially fatal to a developing foetus: all these women would be advised against pregnancy.

Both forms of surrogacy offer a man a chance to have a child that is biologically his own, but they will be of less help to couples where there is a male factor problem contributing to their infertility. However, this problem can be overcome if the couple are contemplating host surrogacy, as the eggs can be inseminated directly with sperm (ICSI). (See p. 132 for further information.)

Surrogacy and the law

Surrogacy is legal in the UK, although it is banned in many countries. The main proviso is that no fee can be paid, and no money other than 'reasonable expenses' can be paid to the surrogate. The reasonable expenses are decided between the intended parents and the surrogate. It is, however, illegal to advertise for surrogates in the UK, or for a surrogate to advertise.

Currently, surrogacy agreements are not considered legally binding on either side. The intended parents cannot establish their rights to the baby before the birth, even when, as in host surrogacy, the baby is genetically related to both intended parents and not the surrogate. The arrangements are therefore largely based on trust.

Surrogacy is not regulated in the same way as other forms of assisted conception, though many people feel it should be brought within the jurisdiction of the HFEA. Intending mothers who are working will find that employment law does not recognise them as being entitled to either maternity leave or maternity pay.

Some couples also consider surrogacy when numerous infertility treatments haven't worked for a combination of reasons, and this seems to be their only chance of parenthood.

Several clinics in the UK will consider gestational surrogacy arrangements for the transfer of embryos derived from the egg and sperm of the intended parents, although they will usually refer each case to their ethics committee for approval.

HOW DOES IT WORK?

If a couple who are infertile seek the help of an agency in finding a surrogate, the usual procedure is for the agency to put some basic non-identifying information about the couple (their first names, ages, height, weight, colouring and so on), and the reason why they are infertile, on a list of couples seeking a surrogate. Once a potential surrogate mother makes contact with the agency, she will see a counsellor to talk through the reasons why she wants to be a surrogate. If all goes well, she is given the list of couples to choose which ones she might be interested in helping. She is then sent further details about them and, if she wishes to meet them, the couple are sent some information about the surrogate. Only after the surrogate and the couple have learned about one another and mutually decided that they wish to meet does the agency provide names and addresses.

Finances

Although a surrogate cannot legally be paid for being a surrogate, she can receive 'reasonable expenses'. There is no strict definition of what these may be, and it is up to the individuals involved to come to an agreement. Any costs incurred by a surrogate directly as a result of the pregnancy would usually be regarded as expenses. In addition, the intended parents may find themselves having to pay for:

- any medical and evaluation tests
- any antenatal care costs
- maternity clothes
- travel costs
- counselling
- legal fees
- insurance
- wages lost as a direct result of the surrogacy

The total cost of a traditional surrogacy will be much lower, since insemination is easier to achieve and does not require the more expensive techniques of IVF procedures.

Whose baby?

Once the baby is born, the intended parents will need to establish their legal parentage. At birth, the baby is registered as the child of the birth mother, whether she is genetically related to the child or not. The father of the child will be registered as the surrogate's husband, if she is married, or her partner, or will be registered as the intended father if the treatment did not take place at a clinic licensed by the HFEA (for example, if the surrogate inseminated herself using the intended father's sperm). If treatment did take place at an HFEA-licensed clinic and the surrogate has no partner, the child is registered as having no legal father.

When the child is six weeks old, the intended parents can apply for a parental order. They will be visited, separately, by a social worker and then the matter will go to court. A parental order will give the couple full and permanent parental rights over the child.

Other issues

In addition to the financial aspects, other decisions will need to be agreed by both the surrogate and intended parents at an early stage. Although some of the areas are uncomfortable, it's preferable to talk over all the implications in detail before entering into a surrogacy arrangement rather than be faced with unpleasant consequences. Jayne says,

'If you think about all these things first, it's much more likely that it will all work out.'

Will the surrogate be 'screened' in any way?

How do you know that the person you are thinking of using as a surrogate is fit, healthy and not carrying an inheritable disease? Will she have been tested for HIV, hepatitis, cystic fibrosis or rubella? If she has a partner, will he have been screened for HIV? In addition, how do you know she is emotionally strong enough for what she is about to undertake? COTS, for example, require that both surrogates and intended parents see a counsellor/ mediator before going on the 'active list' of Triangle, their off- shoot organisation which puts surrogates and hopeful couples in touch with one another.

How involved will the intended parents be in the pregnancy?

For example, where will the antenatal care take place? Will the intended parents be able to accompany the surrogate to routine antenatal visits? Similarly, everyone involved needs to remember that the surrogate runs all the risks associated with pregnancy and labour, and that problems may occur just as they might in any pregnancy. How will you cope with any medical emergencies?

Should the surrogate have an amniocentesis?

An amniocentesis is often advised, even if the surrogate is young and healthy, as the eggs or sperm may be from an older couple and so there is a greater risk of genetic problems. Whether the surrogate will have an abortion if the baby has a chromosomal abnormality needs to be thoroughly discussed in advance so that, if such an unfortunate outcome occurs, all parties are happy with the decision.

What happens if the child is born with a disability?
There is no guarantee of a 'perfect baby' for anyone, and the parents need to consider this in advance. In surrogacy arrangements, the responsibility for the child generally passes to the intended parents upon birth.

Caveats and recommendations

Surrogacy is a process with few guarantees and certainties. Although a written contract may be in place, case law on what happens when things go wrong in surrogacy arrangements offers intended parents few safeguards, a fact which will make some parents feel more uncomfortable than others. Jayne says,

'Of course surrogacy has its risks, but everything does. And if it had gone wrong, let's face it, we'd be no worse off than we were already.'

If you feel that a surrogacy arrangement would be the right step for you, you should first consult with your health professionals that this is a viable option medically, socially and psychologically. As well as putting the legal safeguards and financial arrangements in place, you need to enlist the help of a surrogate whose aims and motivations chime with your own. Jayne says,

'You need to take your time getting to know her. You're entrusting her with a profound responsibility.'

Despite all these caveats, there's no doubt that, when surrogacy arrangements work well, they do allow couples to have their own child when it would otherwise have been impossible. Jayne says,

'Surrogacy was a big decision to make. But we had tried everything, including trying to adopt. We had been members of COTS for several years, but had decided we would try to adopt first as we thought, "Why create a new life when there are already children waiting for us?" I'd had years of treatment, four goes at IVF – three of which had to be abandoned as they couldn't get the hormones right – and we couldn't have afforded any more IVF, or host surrogacy. When we realised we were getting nowhere with the adoption, this was the only option left.'

Similarly, Marcy, who has had a hysterectomy, was resigned to childlessness until she enquired further into surrogacy.

'I actually thought it was illegal. I hadn't realised what it could offer us.'

WHY WOULD ANYONE BE A SURROGATE?

Sometimes a surrogate will be motivated to help a particular couple and may be a relative or close friend of the intended parents. There are many cases throughout the world where one sister has carried a baby for another who could not. Others find it easier to help someone not known to them, which avoids the potential difficulty of seeing the child frequently.

Most potential surrogates already have their own children, so know how precious children can be. Cathy has just signed with an agency in the USA as a potential surrogate mother:

'I don't know what I would have done if I hadn't been able to have children. My three boys are my whole life. I saw the ad for surrogates and I started talking to my friends about whether this was something they would do. Every one of them had a reason why not. They got sick

in early pregnancy, they were too busy with their own lives, they couldn't get involved. I started thinking, if all these people won't do it, who will? So I thought, if you really want to help these people who can't have children, you should do it yourself.'

Some have seen members of their own family or friends battle against infertility, as Nichole had:

'I got the idea of surrogacy from having relatives who were infertile. I told my husband's brother one day that I would carry a baby for him and his wife. My mother also wanted a baby with the person she was with for six years, but she had her tubes tied. I felt bad for these two particular couples, because I love babies, and believe every couple should share a child together if they so choose, so it made me want to make it possible for them. For one reason or another they didn't choose to go this route, but that's what gave me the idea. Then one day I saw a surrogacy agency ad in the paper. I talked it through with my husband, who supported me from the start. I called the number to ask if they needed a carrier, and 11 months later the agency called me with a couple who wanted to meet us.'

Gill, who has been a surrogate mother for three different couples, admits that her initial motivation was unusual.

'I knew I didn't want children of my own, so being a surrogate was the only way I was ever going to experience pregnancy and giving birth. COTS took a lot of persuading that I could be a surrogate when I'd never had children of my own and had no idea what it would be like, but it was something I was ready for.'

Very rarely is money the main motivating factor. Most surrogates derive a great deal of satisfaction from knowing that they have 'put something positive into the world', as Nichole phrases it, and literally made a dream come true. Gill found that, the first time around,

'The idea that I'd be getting money made me really embarrassed. The second time I knew what I'd be going through, so I had no problems accepting the expenses. I earn that money and more for the wear and tear on my body and the risk to my health. I could have got pre-eclampsia and died, for heaven's sake.'

Yet even in the USA, where commercial surrogacy is legal and more common, a surrogate may find that her own friends and family don't easily accept the role the woman wants to take on, as Nichole found:

'Once my husband and I agreed we both wanted to do this, we shared it with our family. The rest of the family was torn. Some supported us and some didn't. Some thought we should get more money, but we weren't in it for the money. Some thought we could get stuck with someone else's babies. There were a lot of mixed feelings in the family and amongst friends. But we were the only ones who mattered in the decision-making.'

Jayne's thoughts are very similar:

'As far as we're concerned, we're very happy with the decision we made to have our baby through surrogacy, and if other people aren't, that's their problem.'

Even so, taking on something which you know some people will oppose or disapprove of does demand strength as well as altruism. This is why most agencies evaluate potential surrogate mothers carefully and insist that they have counselling before committing themselves to the physical and emotional stresses they will un-doubtedly encounter. When Jayne and Mark were considering surrogates they met the surrogates' families as well.

'It was very reassuring to know that their families supported them. If they'd had any doubts, then it was much more likely that the surrogate would come to have doubts, too.'

WHAT HAPPENS?

There are certain stages that all parties in the process must go through, and the social and psychological pressures will be different throughout a pregnancy in which the woman carrying the baby is not its intended parent. Choosing which couples the surrogate would be most willing to help can take a while. Jayne says,

'Within two weeks of us going on the lists, a surrogate chose us. She was 35, so I felt there was more of a risk of Down's, and she had only had one child, so we didn't feel she really suited us. Another surrogate chose us and we found out that she had had three boys. We thought, "What if she has a girl?" It might be harder for her to part with a girl. We also knew that we would prefer a surrogate who was already married or in a relationship, so that her life wasn't so likely to change, and so that the four of us could go out together as couples.'

Laura, the surrogate who eventually had a baby girl for Jayne and Mark, already had two children of her own. Although she definitely didn't want any more, she loved being pregnant, had already been a surrogate mother for another couple and had been a foster mother.

All these factors influenced Jayne's choice.

'She knew what it was like to give up a child – that was the main thing. This is not to say things wouldn't have worked out with the other surrogate mothers, but we felt it best to reduce all the possible risk factors.'

It was very important to Gill that the couples she was assisting really needed help.

'They had been through everything. Their only option was surrogacy. With one couple, for example, she had been pregnant but her uterus had ruptured in labour and the baby had died. Knowing things like

that made it far more than a "business arrangement", although there have to be elements of that, too.'

Meeting

The initial meeting can be stressful, but occasionally everyone knows it's going to work. Gill says,

'With my first couple, we hit it off right away. And you have to "hit it off". You are embarking on a relationship that will last not only for the 18 months or so it usually takes from the initial meeting to the birth of a baby, but, in one way or another, for the rest of your lives.'

As Gill remarks, she felt that one of her couples was quite relieved at the initial meeting 'to find that surrogates are quite normal people'.
  Nichole remembers:

'Our first meeting with the parents was nerve-racking, but beautiful. We met at the house of the woman who runs the agency. The couple brought me a dozen white roses. We spent a couple of hours chatting and getting to know each other and sharing our feelings around all of it. We were all very honest about what we would like out of it before, during and after the birth/pregnancy. We left each other all feeling nervous. Because they then decide if they like us. If they do, they call the agency, who then calls us, and we tell the woman whether we want to or not. Only if both sides say yes do we then call each other direct.'

Jayne strongly believes that, for surrogacy to work, the surrogate and her partner and the couple must become friends first.

'It's quite strange when you first meet, as it's like going on a blind date. Within a couple of meetings you click, or not, as you would do with any partner. You must have more than a baby in common.'

Deciding to go ahead

Jayne says,

'We met Laura and within a couple of months knew that she was right for us, and she decided she did want to help us to have a child. COTS recommend that you wait between three and six months before starting to try for pregnancy, but we were so confident we went ahead sooner. Another factor behind this decision is that my mother was terminally ill. My parents met Laura, and three months later my mum died. I like to think she died knowing this was going to work for us.'

Nichole admits that the final decision needed careful consideration.

'When the couple chose us, my husband felt a little nervous about how I would feel after the birth, or carrying someone else's baby. He wasn't so sure I would feel good after leaving the baby. But we talked a lot, and he eventually agreed that I felt strong enough.'

Sharing the news

Not everyone will 'go public' with their surrogacy arrangements, though total secrecy is obviously impossible. Gill kept the fact that she was a surrogate a secret from the hospital staff during her labour for her first two surrogacies, which caused some problems, especially with the second.

'They knew it was my second baby, and I was worried that if he cried they'd think I would know what to do – and of course I didn't.'

She changed her mind for the third.

'Everybody knew that time that I was a surrogate and it was so nice to be able to be honest. They put me in a room on my own after the birth, took the baby away to the nursery. It was so much better. But I could

only do that because I'm a different person now than the person I was when I first became a surrogate. I'm so much more confident and not afraid of other people's reactions.'

Not everyone might go as far as Gill and the intended parents did the third time, however, as she was filmed by a BBC documentary crew handing over the baby to his parents.

Nevertheless, both the surrogate and the intended parents will inevitably meet some negative reactions although Nichole found that

'After the pregnancy was in progress, the negative people came around to understanding.'

But it's not always so easy. Jayne knew that some people were against what she was doing,

'They'd say things like "I think a woman would be emotionally damaged by giving up a child," but giving a wanted child to a couple who very much want a baby is not the same as giving a child up for adoption. In surrogacy, the child is being conceived on purpose. Many children who are adopted will feel abandoned, but a surrogate's child will always know it was wanted.'

Gill thinks that too many people still think of surrogacy in purely business terms.

'It's not just a commercial contract. Those couples will always be my friends, because I've got to know them. If you were doing it just for money, the money would not be enough. You have to want to do it in your heart.'

Jayne found that many of her friends and relatives were worried about it all going wrong.

'It can be worrying if all you've heard about it is what you read in the press. Everyone thought Mark and I were very "brave" to contemplate surrogacy in case the surrogacy went wrong or the surrogate could not give up the baby. But I knew that in reality only about 3 per cent of arrangements do fall through, and when things do go wrong there are usually reasons to explain why. When you look into it, you find that adoption has a higher failure rate, with the number of adoptions that fall through.'

Conception

Most surrogacies are still done in the traditional way – the surrogate inseminates herself with the father's semen around the time she is ovulating. Conception probably won't happen the first time. Gill used ovulation predictor kits to work out when she was ovulating, but even so

'It took seven months with my first couple, then three, which was very quick, and then five, although that seemed to be going on forever. I got very frustrated that I wasn't getting pregnant.'

Jayne says,

'I don't think the insemination needs to be done in a hospital. Laura used OPKs to work out when she was ovulating, and we would go round to her house, have a chat, have a cup of tea, play with the children and then Mark would go upstairs to produce a sample. Laura always made him feel very comfortable about it, and he didn't find it too embarrassing as he'd done it on so many occasions at the hospital. Then later Laura inseminated herself with a syringe. We did this about three times each cycle.'

Gill, too, found the process quite simple, although she was nervous the first few times. She describes a typical situation:

*'I went up to stay with them when it was round about the right time.
We always went out to dinner or somewhere, then we'd go back to their
house. When I was in bed, the father would come in with a little pot
containing the semen and give it to me. I kept it under my arm for a little
while, until it went runny, then I'd put it inside me, put my bum up on
pillows for an hour or so, then turn over and go to sleep.'*

Nichole has a different perspective because she was a gestational
carrier.

*'The egg transfer was nice. The couple's eggs and sperm were joined and
made into embryos, which sat in a dish for three days (as they would
have inside the body). Then I was given Valium to relax my body. My
legs were up in stirrups. They put the embryos into me, four of them,
and I lay with my legs up for two hours. Then I went home on bed rest
for four days so the embryos would attach to my uterus. (I had been on
different medications for three months prior, which tricked my body into
thinking it was pregnant.) The doctors did a pregnancy test on day 12,
which showed high readings. So we had a feeling there were at least
two. The parents were really nervous. I went for an ultrasound at two to
three weeks pregnant and we saw two sacs. Two out of the four eggs had
implanted the first time. The parents were so excited. They were also
nervous, because they had no kids and now they were going to have
two.'*

Waiting to find out whether the surrogate is pregnant can be a very
tense time. Jayne says,

*'I was always shaking when the phone rang. In the end I had to get
Caller Display as I answered every call with such anticipation. It took
six months to work, and by then we were all getting disheartened.
Laura needed comforting just as much as we did when she wasn't
pregnant and was beginning to feel that she was letting us down. She
normally conceives on the first or second month of trying, and ended up
going to the doctor's as she was sure she had become infertile! The*

doctor sent her to hospital for a scan to see if she was ovulating properly, as her cycles had become very irregular. The plan was to put her on a mild fertility drug, as it was becoming very difficult to know when ovulation was going to be – but we never had to do that in the end, as she conceived that very month. I can't tell you the joy that we felt. We were thrilled.'

Pregnancy

Most people expect a surrogate to feel very differently about the pregnancy from how she would if she was giving birth to a child whom she intended to keep, but Nichole found that she didn't.

'Actually I felt like I should be more careful, and more responsible, so I would do a great job for these people and then if anything went wrong with the babies I would know I did the best I could. It was like babysitting in a sense. I had to protect these babies almost better than my own, because these people trusted me to do so.'

Gill enjoyed being pregnant.

'I love it, absolutely love it, feeling the baby move around – all of that. I miss it.'

With the first two couples for whom Gill carried a child, the surrogacy was kept secret, so the parents were not able to participate in any of the antenatal care; but with the third they were. Jayne felt very involved in her surrogate's pregnancy:

'It was wonderful going through the pregnancy with Laura, and I didn't feel at all jealous as I have done when friends and relatives got pregnant. At 12 weeks, we had our first scan. It was a wonderful feeling to see our baby waving back at us. We had two further scans during the pregnancy, because the doctors thought Abigail was a little on the small side. Apart from that, we had no real problems apart from

a scare at 32 weeks when Laura had an antenatal check and the heartbeat was slow. We had to wait 24 hours for Laura to have a detailed scan – and then we found that the baby had been asleep! We were all very relieved. I can't say it was just like being pregnant ourselves, but it was very, very close. Whenever Laura talked about the baby it was always "our baby", not "my baby". And she sent me a Mother's Day card. She did everything to make it something special for me.'

The parents of the twins Nicole gave birth to were also closely involved:

'We agreed from Day 1 that we wanted the parents to come to every appointment, and every ultrasound, and the birth. They agreed that they wanted to, too. So unless weather prevented them from driving the two hours, they came to every appointment, ultrasound, egg-transfer and the birth of their babies. It was beautiful!'

The birth

Jayne recalls,

'Finally the day came when Abigail was going to be born. Laura phoned to say her waters had broken, but when we arrived at the hospital contractions had stopped. We stayed a while with Laura, then went to Laura's mum's house to await further news. Just before midnight, the hospital rang to say we should come over as Laura was now in labour. I was allowed into the labour room with Laura and the midwife. Mark preferred to wait outside – he feels faint just watching Casualty! At 1.44a.m. our beautiful daughter Abigail Laura was born. Laura asked if I would like to cut the cord, which I did; then Abigail was handed straight to me. Mark then came in and held our daughter and marvelled at her. We then handed Abigail to Laura for her to hold. Lots of photographs were taken.'

Nichole says,

'I had believed I would feel somewhat detached at the birth, because I knew they weren't my eggs and the babies wouldn't even resemble me, but I was just as involved as with my own children.'

The intended parents were with Nichole to see their twins born, but not all parents are. Sometimes this is down to the circumstances of the birth itself. Gill says,

'I wanted a water birth, but it takes 20 minutes to fill the pool and 25 minutes to heat it, and I was only in hospital 17 minutes before Jamie arrived. The parents could never have driven there in time.'

Her own parents were there, however.

'It was the right thing for me not to have the parents at the birth. I just wanted my mum. I had to prise Jamie away from my father in the end. He gave me a cuddle afterwards and said how proud he was of me. Giving birth is my last real link to the child. The parents are going to have that child for the rest of their lives, but it's the last moment of that special relationship for me. And when the baby's born, it's like you're in shock. There's no immediate rush of emotion, apart from being relieved the pain has finally stopped. The emotion came later, usually after I'd finished being stitched up.'

And there are emotions, too. When Gill had her first baby for another couple, the little girl was delivered after a difficult labour.

'She was whimpering and I found it very upsetting that she was crying. I felt an overwhelming protectiveness towards her, like I'd never felt in my whole life. I didn't love her, didn't want to take her home with me, but I did want to protect her. So where do all these feelings go?'

Jayne found the hospital staff very understanding and supportive of her surrogacy arrangement.

'They were wonderful. After Abigail was born, Laura was given a room of her own in the antenatal ward so she didn't have to be surrounded by other people's babies, and they provided a family room for Abigail, Mark and me. A nurse bathed Abigail, and then Mark and I both took it in turns to feed her.'

Handing the baby over

Jayne remembers with fondness the day they left hospital:

'In the morning, Laura's mum came to the hospital to take her home. Before they left, Laura's mum and Laura's children visited Abigail. We left the hospital in the afternoon, after our parentcraft classes.'

After Gill had been discharged from the hospital with her first baby – the staff there had not known it was a surrogate birth – she met the couple at her parents' house.

'My mum brought the baby downstairs and handed her to her new mother. They stayed a couple of hours. It was a very emotional time. I cried, everyone cried. I still cry sometimes when I think about it.'

Nichole admits,

'I was sadly surprised at how difficult it was when it was time to leave the hospital. It really wasn't so much "handing the babies over" because the parents stayed in a motel near the hospital for the four days that I was there, and we were together for most of that time. The sadness came from the whole thing ending. I was going to miss hearing from the parents every day, miss being pregnant with two babies kicking, miss seeing my doctor, miss the anticipation of it all, miss the year of constant happenings surrounding the pregnancy, and miss

the babies when I went home empty-handed. Saying goodbye was tear-jerking for everyone. I cried, they cried, my mum cried! It was very sad. Watching them drive away with the babies was so sad – I felt very left out.'

Gill remembers that the couple for whom she had her first baby had to stop to buy a baby car seat on the way down to collect their daughter.

'That was how much they didn't trust me. Not in a nasty way, but I know they didn't want to let themselves hope too much, just in case I didn't hand the baby over.'

The next two babies Gill had were both boys and, for her, this made it easier to part with them.

'They were so obviously their father's sons. I know if the last one had been a girl, I'd have had more problems handing her over.'

Afterwards

The parents have the joy of their baby. For most couples, this will be the baby they thought they could never have, and now they will be taking their little bundle home feeling that they have experienced a miracle.

But what about the surrogate? Gill says,

'You do get depressed afterwards, and it's mainly because your hormones are all over the place. Even though you've always known that you're going to give away the baby, your body has still been preparing you to look after something. I was depressed for about six months after the birth each time. It's not depression from giving up the child, because never for one second had I ever considered the child mine, but it's from the hormones being out of place.'

Nichole found that:

'Post-partum depression was not so bad after the twins. It was more of an empty feeling. I was missing the parents, the babies, the doctors, the phone calls, the excitement and anticipation . . . But my family was so supportive, I got through it really well. I also had a therapist whom I spoke to weekly. Since then I have had my own baby, my fifth and last baby, who is now six months old.'

Keeping in touch

After the baby is born, some surrogates and parents will gradually drift apart, others will make a decision to go their separate ways, perhaps because they don't want the child to grow up confused, and yet others will stay closely in touch. Keeping in touch isn't an option that everyone will pursue, but when it does happen it can bring a lot of joy. Gill says,

'It was hard, with my first couple, to know how much contact to have with the child afterwards. It's taken us years to work out how we stand. But the whole basis of the relationship is that you have to be honest with each other, so you have to say what you do and do not want.'

There's often a gap between the birth and the resumption of contact, while everyone adjusts to the new situation. Gill says,

'I actually didn't want to see the family for the first four or five months after the birth. I needed time to get myself back to myself. I saw them at three weeks to register the birth, but then not for another few months.'

Nichole, too, stopped hearing from her family for a while, but puts this down to the fact that they were now having to cope with life with twins.

'Once the parents got semi-adjusted to having two babies, I began to hear from them a lot. We're still in touch, even though the babies I had for them are two years old now. The parents call me and send pictures. They just sent a big 8 × 10 picture of them for my birthday. We used to visit a lot, but they moved out of Massachusetts to Connecticut, so we haven't driven there yet – but we will.'

Nearly two years after Abigail's birth, says Jayne,

'We still keep in touch with Laura. All she expected from us initially in the form of contact was news on how Abigail was growing up, and pictures at least once a year. Some people are surprised that we still see her – but why not? We've become such good friends that we see each other as often as good friends would. We talk on the phone, meet every few months, send her pictures of Abigail. We also invited her to Abigail's christening and will invite her to Abigail's wedding, should she get married in the future. I don't feel threatened by Laura, and she doesn't interfere with the way I bring up Abigail. When she holds Abigail, I can see the joy in her face in bringing such a wanted baby into the world who is so loved by her parents.'

Telling the surrogate child

The general consensus seems to be that secrecy isn't the best policy. COTS, for example, won't support any couple through a surrogacy arrangement unless they are prepared to tell the child about his or her origins. Once a child reaches the age of 18, he or she will be able to obtain a copy of the original birth certificate – which will, of course, include the name of the surrogate mother. Anyone asking for this information, which also has a cross-reference to the Parental Order Register, will be offered counselling, but it must surely be in the child's best interests that the news of the surrogacy doesn't come as a shock.

Gill, who has kept in touch with all three families, feels that it will be easier for them to tell the child *'because I won't be a stranger when the child is told. I don't think you can force an explanation on them, but they absorb more than we think they do. I think they will gradually get to know.'*

Jayne keeps a picture book with all the family's photographs in.

'There's a picture of me holding Abigail in the hospital, and one of Mark, and one of Laura, "Auntie Laura". Abigail doesn't know yet quite how she fits in, but we've made her aware of Laura from the start. As she grows up, Abigail will be told how she was born and who her birth mother is. She'll be told that Laura carried her in her tummy because I have a broken tummy. When she's old enough to understand about genetics, she'll then be told that Laura also provided the egg and that Laura's children are her biological half-brother and half-sister. Laura's children understand that they have a very special sister and are very proud of their mum for helping us. I'm sure Abigail will feel the same when she grows up.'

IS SURROGACY RIGHT FOR US?

Naturally, those for whom surrogacy has worked are fervent proselytisers on the topic. Jayne says,

'We tried for years and years to have a child, and surrogacy made our dream come true. Not only have we been blessed with a wonderful baby, but we have made a friend for life. Abigail is a wonderful, happy toddler. My heart melts every time she smiles at me and calls me Mummy.'

Jayne believes it's an option people should consider despite the unwillingness of many in the medical profession to countenance it as a good way forward.

'Some doctors won't do host or IVF surrogacy until you've done "enough" IVF treatments of your own to prove it won't work. But

think of the trauma that that would do to your mind and body. I can't thank Laura enough for what she's done for us. She's made our lives have substance and meaning.'

But things don't go so well every time. Katy is currently pregnant for a couple whom she liked a great deal initially, but it hasn't been the experience she hoped for.

'I'm sad. I just don't get on with them when it comes down to it. I wouldn't dream of keeping the baby, but they've expressed disappointment that it's a boy and not a girl, for example – things like that. You read about surrogates letting couples down, but sometimes couples can let surrogates down, too.'

There can be huge upsets along the way, too, but this is hardly surprising when everyone is testing the boundaries of new relationships. Gill, who wanted to take drugs to stop her breastmilk coming in, lost her temper when she was asked to express milk for one couple.

'I was very angry because I had made it clear what I wanted, but this was being disregarded. I felt like I was expected to act like a cow.'

Eventually the issue was resolved, but it shows how deep the trust between all the parties needs to be.
    Jayne says,

'There are always tensions and relationship problems within families, so you must expect some in a relationship like this, too, and work through them. Not a day goes by when Mark and I don't tell ourselves how lucky we are. All those years of infertility and hoping are firmly in the past. I am making the most of every day and enjoying every minute. Motherhood is everything I expected it to be and more.'

In fact Laura intended to have a second child for Jayne and Mark, but circumstances conspired against this:

'Just as we started trying for our second child, Laura met a wonderful man and is now getting married later this year. Although she was prepared to continue and her husband-to-be was happy for her to continue, we all decided, after a lot of thought, that it was not to be – not to mention the fact that our surrogate mother would look pretty strange getting married when she was eight months pregnant! We totally understand, and wish her all the best for the future.'

Jayne is also looking to the future herself.

'We've been lucky enough to meet another wonderful surrogate mother. I thought no one would choose us again, having already achieved parenthood, but our new surrogate mother has already expressed an interest in having a third child for us if all goes well. It took ten years to have just one child, and we might finally be parents of three in the end.'

There is no doubt that more and more couples are considering surrogacy as a way of having their family. Since the agency was set up on Mothering Sunday 1988, COTS have experienced a dramatic rise in enquiries and births. In the beginning, when they first started putting surrogates and couples in touch with one another, there were one or two births a year. In 1997, they were involved in 41. They estimate that they send out about a thousand booklets a year to couples considering surrogacy, although not everyone follows that up. It is clear, however, that more and more couples are doing so.

The last word goes to Jayne:

'We are a family at long last. The wait has been worth it.'

8

Miscarriage

Miscarriage can be one of the most devastating and over-whelming experiences a couple will ever face. The sense of grief and sadness can persist for many months. It is with some initial disbelief, therefore, that many couples find that this trauma in their lives is considered by the medical profession as no more than 'bad luck'.

In many ways, the experts are right. For most women, most of the time, miscarriage *is* just bad luck. There is always the chance that any pregnancy will end with a miscarriage: as many as one in five miscarry in the normal course of events, sometimes so early that the woman may scarcely have suspected she was pregnant, only wondering when she has a slightly later and heavier period. The main cause of miscarriage seems to be a chromosomal abnormality in the developing embryo, stemming from the time of conception. It is therefore nature's way of ensuring that only embryos with a good chance of being healthy are carried to term. Around a quarter of all women who become pregnant will experience a miscarriage at some point, but knowing that this is the most common complication of pregnancy doesn't alleviate the pain when it happens.

WHAT HAPPENS?

Miscarriages usually start with the loss of small amounts of blood, though before this you may feel some cramps or aches. Feeling that a miscarriage is about to happen is stressful on both the physical and emotional level. Helia, who had a miscarriage at seven weeks following IVF treatment, did what many women instinctively do:

'I went straight to bed and stayed there, although I knew from my reading that staying in bed wouldn't make any difference one way or the other. I felt a strong need, though, to put all my energies into sustaining the pregnancy, and if that meant doing nothing, then that was what I was going to do.'

Sadly, as Helia knew, there seems to be very little that can prevent a pregnancy from miscarrying once it has begun to do so.

ECTOPIC PREGNANCY

When an embryo implants elsewhere than in the uterus, most often in one of the fallopian tubes, it won't be able to develop normally as there isn't enough space for it to grow and there is no endometrium to nourish it. An ectopic pregnancy can have serious consequences for a woman because it causes internal bleeding. If an ectopic is suspected it's essential that it's identified early, and it will always need removing immediately. This is done either by surgery, which may lead to further damage or complete removal of the tube, or with an injection of methotrexate if the ectopic is discovered early enough, after which it will slowly absorb into the body.

Equally sadly, a miscarriage is something that many women feel health professionals still don't seem to understand. Gail felt, when she ended up in hospital, 'that I might as well have gone to have my appendix out'. She had to telephone her partner in the middle of the night just to get him to come and be with her for emotional support. As she went to the bathroom and bled all over the floor, a nurse came along and told her to get back into bed because she was making a mess. Gail remembers,

'I thought, "That's not a mess, that's my baby. I don't want to be losing my baby all over the floor like this." But no one could understand that.'

Perhaps because medical staff know that most women who miscarry go on to be pregnant again within a few months, they have a perspective on your situation which you, in your distress, cannot have.

A pregnancy loss that occurs after a long period of trying for a baby can be extremely traumatic – another hurt and disappointment after possibly years of sadness and the first chances of hope; yet the risks of this happening are, unfortunately, higher than average. Women with partially blocked tubes are more prone to ectopics, and IVF pregnancies are more likely to result in an ectopic than are spontaneous pregnancies. In addition an older woman, who may have undergone several years of infertility treatments, is at greater risk of miscarriage because, as she grows older, the eggs that her ovaries produce are more likely to contain chromosomal abnormalities.

Mary miscarried twins at 17 weeks and the feelings of loss went very deep:

'As we walked through the hospital corridors on the way home, I thought of all the clothes I'd bought them that they'd never wear. This time we'd seemed so close, I'd begun to believe that they really would be born. I couldn't bear to open the chest of drawers where I'd put those clothes, but I'd think about them, knowing they were there. And as the months went on and we just didn't conceive again, I had to ask Kevin to take them away and give them to a charity shop. I couldn't look at them or touch them myself.'

Hilary has had two miscarriages, the latest a year ago when she lost the baby at 19 weeks.

'The doctors thought that fibroids might be causing implantation problems and I've had treatment for this, but I'm 43 now and think

*that the chances of conceiving again are very small, even though we've
now been offered GIFT.'*

Grieving for a baby who has been lost, whether through an ectopic,
miscarriage, stillbirth or death, is a long and painful process, but a
necessary one. No baby you ever go on to have will be a substitute
for the lost baby. You may feel that you need a long time to come to
terms with the loss of your baby before you go on to try infertility
treatment again. And in the meantime you will *still* have to deal
with everyone who does the equivalent of pat you on the head and
tell you, 'Never mind. At least you know you can get pregnant
again.'

RECURRENT MISCARRIAGE

A miscarriage, however agonising, does indicate that a couple can
conceive, and the chances are that next time, without any specific
treatment, they will go on to have a normal pregnancy and a
healthy baby. But when one miscarriage is followed by a second,
and perhaps another, this is a sign that there may be something
wrong rather than just 'bad luck'.

Recurrent miscarriage is defined as the loss of three or more
consecutive pregnancies. Sometimes these will happen after spontaneous conception; at other times they will happen when the
couple have already been undergoing some form of infertility
treatment.

Possible causes

Tests can now be carried out to try to determine the reason for
recurrent miscarriage, and your doctor may feel that it is worth
initiating some of these if you have had two miscarriages. If an
underlying condition is found, treatment to solve the particular
problem may be possible, increasing the chances that a pregnancy
can be carried to term. You need to remember, however, that a

cause for recurrent miscarriage, typically one of those listed below, can only be clearly identified in a very small percentage of women. Most of the time, sadly, no cause can be found.

- *raised antiphospholipid antibodies:* antiphospholipid antibody syndrome (APS; see p. 200) is a disorder of the immune system which can cause recurrent miscarriage and this can be tested for
- *chromosome problems:* as individuals neither parent has a problem, but any resulting embryo has a high risk of abnormality
- *physical abnormalities in the uterus:* an unusually shaped womb may present problems with implantation; this can be congenital or caused by the growth of fibroids
- *cervical incompetence:* a weakness in the cervix may cause miscarriage, as the baby grows and develops, after the twelfth week or so of pregnancy
- *polycystic ovary syndrome:* while PCOS often means a couple will have trouble conceiving at all, studies show that a woman with PCOS and raised levels of luteinising hormone runs an increased risk of miscarriage
- *other immunological factors*: rarely, some couples have similar components in their immune systems, with the result that the woman's body rejects rather than accepts the pregnancy; the immune disease systemic lupus erythematosus is also associated with miscarriage; and there are other immune disorders which might be tested for

People have tried to prevent recurrent miscarriage, not always with happy results. In the USA between the 1950s and 1970s some women were given DES (diethyl stilboestrol), a synthetic hormone. However, it was found that children born after DES treatment often had infertility problems themselves.

Far from becoming desensitised, many parents find that each miscarriage is just as painful as the first, as Bernadette did:

'I've actually become pregnant five times in the past six years. I'm lucky – I have one beautiful daughter, Celine, to show for it. But my other four pregnancies ended in a miscarriage. My last miscarriage was just over a year ago, when I was 39. We've decided that we were meant only to have Celine, so we've now stopped trying to get pregnant again. The pain and the hope each time were just too much to bear.'

After Sally had her son, Ben, she had a great deal of difficulty conceiving again, even though she was prescribed drugs to help her ovulate.

'I was eventually given a lap and dye which showed pelvic scarring. Three years after Ben had been born, I had a miscarriage at six weeks. The next year an ectopic, then later that year another miscarriage. The next year I had another miscarriage at six weeks. Our GP suggested we try IVF, even though I didn't feel that getting pregnant was the problem – the problem was carrying. We then found out that a hospital in London was carrying out research into similar cases, investigating a possible immune problem. They took us on for treatment and I was injected with Jack's white blood cells to build up immunity. Our daughter was born a year later.'

Progesterone levels

In pregnancies which end in miscarriage, the levels of pro-gesterone are sometimes found to be low. This led, at one time, to progesterone supplements being given as a preven-tative measure, but these have been shown to be of no clinical benefit and don't increase the likelihood of a pregnancy continuing. Progesterone supplements are indeed needed when a couple have conceived through IVF, as the usual support mechanisms from the corpus luteum are not present. Low progesterone levels after unassisted conception are now thought to reflect the fact that an early pregnancy is failing rather than being the cause of the miscarriage.

New hope with heparin?

Antiphospholipid antibody syndrome (APS) has been the focus of much recent research. It's caused when a person's immune system produces a type of antibody that acts against the body itself rather than against a germ or viral infection. A woman with APS may never know she has the condition because it doesn't make you feel unwell, but it's associated with recurrent miscarriage and you can have a blood test to check for this.

Around 15 per cent of women suffering recurrent miscarriage are found to have persistently high levels of antiphospholipid antibodies in their blood. It's thought that this might lead to miscarriage because a thrombosis (blood clot) forms in the developing links between the uterus and the placenta, although doctors still don't know exactly how the antibodies affect pregnancy. Under normal circumstances, the chances for such women of a pregnancy succeeding without any intervention are only around 10 per cent. It's been known for a while that taking a low dose of aspirin can increase the chances of success for these women, but a recent study, carried out at the specialist recurrent miscarriage clinic at St Mary's Hospital in London, found that the addition of heparin injections to the use of aspirin further improved the live birth rate for pregnant women with antiphospholipid antibodies.[7]

The women in the study were divided into two groups, with 45 women in each, and given either just aspirin or aspirin combined with self-administered heparin injections. There were 32 live births in the aspirin-plus-heparin group, compared to 19 in the aspirin-only group. There were still some problems later in the pregnancy for some women: of the 51 successful pregnancies, 12 were delivered before 37 weeks (because of premature labour, growth retardation in the foetus or pre-eclampsia), so the rigours of careful monitoring were essential. All the babies were fine.

The authors do point out that these women were patients at a highly specialised recurrent miscarriage clinic and they received extensive support and monitoring throughout their pregnancies, so it may be difficult for other clinics to achieve similar levels of success. Nevertheless, as the authors point out, 'Although such women represent less than 20 per cent of all sufferers of recurrent miscarriage, they are easily identified, and any advance in the management of such a distressing condition is to be welcomed.'

It is only recently that antiphospholipid antibodies were discovered and their significance understood, so the information available for doctors to work with is limited, but more research and studies are being carried out around the world. More and more research is also being done into other immunological factors, such as antithyroid antibodies (where a woman produces antibodies to her own thyroid gland), that seem to prevent the successful implantation and development of the embryo either after a spontaneous conception or IVF.

9

Secondary Infertility

'Secondary' infertility is often defined as 'the inability to conceive after giving birth to at least one child'. This may be one reason why many couples with secondary infertility feel that they elicit much less sympathy, both from ordinary people and from the medical profession, than those who can't conceive at all. Yet there are also couples with secondary infertility who have lost their first child through miscarriage or death, and people who have a 'first' family and find it difficult to start a second with a new partner. Nobody knows how widespread a problem secondary infertility is, because many couples affected by it will never seek medical help.

Sometimes the experience of secondary infertility can be an even more unexpected blow to the couple than the idea of not having a child at all, as Sue explains.

'We just assumed it would be easy for us to have another child. After all, we'd already had one baby so we knew everything worked. It came as a big shock to be told that it wasn't likely we would conceive again.'

Most parents expect to have more than one child. There are some who choose to have just one, but most of us, when we have our first child, are already conscious of the process of building a family in which that child will one day have a sibling.

A couple's natural fertility decreases with age, and therefore their chances of success in conceiving are always less second time around. However, where couples have been investigated for secondary infertility problems, the causes turn out to be almost identical to those for couples experiencing primary infertility – sperm defects, ovulation failure, tubal damage and endometriosis. Some research has suggested that damage caused by infection at the time of the previous birth or miscarriage, or from an ectopic pregnancy, can increase the likelihood of secondary infertility.

It was only when Sue went for routine tests and investigations, after four years of trying for a second child, that she and her partner Colin discovered why it might have taken them three years to conceive without intervention the first time round.

'We discovered that Colin had a low sperm count, and the post-coital test showed that I had hostile mucus as well.'

Lena has been taking drugs to help her ovulate for the past year, but still isn't pregnant.

'Like everyone else, we just assumed it would happen when we started treatment. I'm 39 this year and resigning myself to the fact that it probably won't happen, but the whole experience has been very traumatic.'

WHO CAN YOU TELL?

Dileni found the depth of her emotions hard to bear, and couldn't share them with anyone. She thought they would feel she was just being 'dramatic' when she already had one healthy baby, after all:

'I had overwhelming happiness that Alexi was here, but the pain of longing for a second baby was at times so intense, the anger and bitterness so great, I felt it consumed me. And yet I was one of the lucky

ones – a fact I reminded myself of daily. I hope this made me a better parent than I might otherwise have been – the one small positive in this sea of negatives.'

Couples who already have one child often experience feelings of frustration, grief and powerlessness when they don't conceive just as intensely as couples with primary infertility, and yet, like Dileni, find this harder to share. Philippa says,

'I feel very alone with this, and it's hard to find people to talk to about it because they don't know what to say to me. They can't say they're sorry for me because I've already got Emily. And yet they can't just dismiss my problem, either.'

The extra pressures of secondary infertility

- society often expects you to have a second child, which may make you feel more worried when you don't
- parents may feel intimidated about seeking treatment for something that might not be perceived as a priority
- health professionals or infertile couples may make parents feel guilty for wanting more children
- the desire for a second or third child may be even stronger than for the first, perhaps because you have experienced parenthood or perhaps because you have had the sadness of losing a baby
- couples may well be older than those who have primary infertility, and awareness of declining fertility may lead to increased stress

---

WHEN YOU HAVE ONE CHILD

Barbara says,

'I know I should be grateful for the fact that I have one child at all, but the urge to have another baby is just as strong as it was when we were trying for Chris. It's not like wanting a new table or a bigger house. It's not something that's rational. And these aren't feelings that you can turn on and off like a tap.'

Philippa agrees:

'When my period arrives I'm just as disappointed as I always used to be when I didn't have a child. People do say to me not to be upset, as if I shouldn't have these feelings, but I do.'

Secondary infertility brings its own additional psychological stresses. Barbara's son Chris, now five, came along without any problems, but a second baby just 'hasn't happened'. Barbara has become very involved as an organiser for her local National Childbirth Trust group, which meant that she was mixing far more in the world of parents, babies and toddlers than she had when she was working.

'People are always asking us when we're going to have the next, and I find it difficult to answer because I just don't know. In the meantime, I see other people who were in my antenatal group go on to have their second, or their third, and I feel I'm being left behind.'

Philippa says,

'I'm jealous, I admit it. I sometimes get a bit resentful when other parents find they have a second on the way very easily, especially when they aren't 100 per cent happy about it.'

Once you have had a child, you may find that you suddenly know lots more people with young children than you used to, simply because you make friends with them when your first child is born. Philippa says,

'It felt like a myth I'd always heard was coming true. There really did seem to be pregnant women everywhere.'

Nurseries and playgroups will bring you in contact with even more, until it seems like the whole world is having families but you are having what people call an 'only child' – which may not be what you wanted. Barbara says,

'People ask me if we've deliberately stopped at one, and I do sense a certain sniffiness when they say this, as if we've done something very selfish or unhealthy.'

Philippa found conflicting feelings within her own family.

'Both my sisters went on to have a second baby not so long after their first. On the one hand they looked at me as if I was doing something unhealthy only having one, and on the other they kept telling me how sensible I was not having another because two were so much work and it was so difficult dealing with two different sets of demands.'

Barbara finally found support through talking to someone at CHILD, one of the national self-help organisations.

'I was talking to the person on the helpline for ages, and as we were talking I found out that she was infertile herself and didn't have children. Immediately I felt awful. I said, "Here am I complaining on and on and you haven't got any children. But she said, "It's how you feel that's important, not what anyone else has or hasn't got." She really understood my feelings, which was wonderful.'

When you already have one child, you might find . . .

- you're more likely to be surrounded by other parents having second or third babies
- you worry about whether your child is missing out because they're an 'only child'
- you're concerned that you're becoming overprotective of your child
- your child may ask why he or she doesn't have a brother or sister
- your beliefs about the optimum age gap between siblings have to be abandoned
- parents may fear that a growing age difference between siblings will mean they will never be close
- you can't find anyone who truly understands what you're going through
- attending an infertility clinic is much more difficult with a child in tow
- finding babysitters so you can have medical treatment can be a problem

---

One factor which you may need to deal with is your child, who may ask, casually or otherwise, whether he or she is going to get a baby brother or sister at some point. Again, the messages can pull you in different directions. Alice found that her daughter, Carrie, started praying for a baby every night.

'All her friends at playgroup had one, and she wanted one, too. She wanted to help out and fetch nappies and help me to bath it – all of those sorts of things. You know the way little girls think of babies as being like dolls. Of course, you can't tell them that the reality is any different. And she seemed to think that not having one was a deliberate fault on our part.'

Sean, on the other hand, told his parents that he didn't want a sibling, of either gender, which made it difficult for Marion when

she needed laser treatment for endometriosis to help her conceive
again.

*'He was very put out that I had to spend time in the hospital and
recovering in bed for something he thought would be a huge disruption
to our cosy family life.'*

If you are diagnosed with a particular infertility problem, you
may find yourselves contemplating treatment which turns out
to be lengthy and expensive. Couples need to consider the
effect of spending time and emotional resources on a subsequent pregnancy, rather than on their first child or children.

Janet and Colin have a son but have had difficulty conceiving
again. She says,

*'We've now spent six years trying for another baby, and ironically I
stopped breastfeeding at five months as I wanted to have the children
close together. We found that Colin had a low sperm count, but
treatment is much more difficult when you already have a child.
We've had two goes at AI with stimulated ovulation on the NHS
and we could have one more try, but I have to get up at 5 a.m. to get to
the hospital for treatment and I think this will be too stressful for us as a
family.'*

Finances can come into it as well, especially if you need an
expensive treatment like IVF. Lucy says,

*'We considered it, but decided that we couldn't afford it. We knew from
experience that it was unlikely to work the first time, and we might need
several attempts, and that kind of financial burden was just too much
when we had Sam's needs to consider.'*

WHEN YOU DON'T HAVE A CHILD

Gilli's experience of secondary infertility began when, after an unplanned but straightforward pregnancy, she and Adam lost their first baby.

'I knew immediately that I wanted another baby. I knew that nothing could or would replace Liam, my beautiful son, but now I knew the wonder of having a child and I longed for another to help fill this terrible void. I was a mother without a child.'

Gilli's periods didn't return for four months:

'I would keep doing pregnancy tests in the vain hope that a blue line would appear, wondering why I didn't become pregnant immediately.'

After her periods had returned and more months went by without her becoming pregnant, Gilli decided to ask her GP if there might be a problem – although she was reassured that she had a good chance of conceiving again because she had already had one child. Tests finally showed that she wasn't ovulating, however, and hormone tablets were prescribed, but without success.

'What was so difficult was the "unknown" aspect of the whole thing. There was no guarantee that I would ever become pregnant again. That fact alone made it hard to carry on with the tablets months after month, but I didn't feel I had much choice. I couldn't find anything that could compensate for not becoming pregnant. I would have suffered virtually anything to have another baby, and at times it felt as though I did.'

OBTAINING TREATMENT

Since secondary infertility is unfortunately sometimes taken less seriously than primary infertility by the medical profession, some couples experience difficulty in obtaining the treatment they feel they need. Isa and Rhodri's first baby, Gwilym, died from Sudden Infant Death syndrome at six weeks of age. After a year of 'nothing happening', Isa went to see her GP:

'He told me that we were probably just trying too hard to replace Gwilym and to relax and give it another year. I started keeping temperature charts, though, and after about six months felt that they showed it was clear I wasn't ovulating. I was then prescribed Clomid and was pregnant in two months.'

Angela has two daughters and feels that no one is taking her desire for more children seriously enough.

'I always wanted four children. We conceived the girls with no problem, but I'm 37 now and we've been trying for three years and I'm worried it just isn't going to happen. I'm on Clomid at the moment, but we haven't been offered any tests. We're told that there can't really be anything wrong with us as we have two children and all we really need to do is relax. . . . Easier said than done. I get the feeling that the medical profession are unwilling to see this as a problem and that we don't rank very high on their list of priorities.'

SUPPORT

It can be harder when you are undergoing treatment for secondary infertility to keep this fact to yourselves. Alison says,

'Peter and I kept having to ask people to have Christopher, and eventually we had to explain to them why. We got away with saying Peter needed check-ups at the hospital for a while, but then, when we

were undergoing the drug treatment and everything and didn't know how long things would take or what time we would be back . . . then we had to tell them the reason.'

There is no doubt that couples with secondary infertility often receive less support than those who are unable to conceive at all, even though their desire for a child may be no less strong than for couples who have never conceived. This in itself makes many couples reluctant to seek treatment.

If you find that people around you cannot understand your feelings, it may help to talk to people in the same situation as yourselves. CHILD and ISSUE (see pp. 278–9) can put you in touch with couples who are having difficulties conceiving following a pregnancy or birth, and there are several newsgroups and mailing lists on the Internet specifically set up as a forum for discussion, sharing information and feelings and providing emotional support for people in this predicament.

Knowing how society expects you to feel cannot change how you do feel. Gilli had an emotional legacy from her 'lost years':

'Of course everyone assumed my problems were over when Callum arrived. Maybe for some people this is so, but after years of treatment, and facing possibly more in the future, I was left with a sense of deep despair.'

Sometimes the discrepancy between the feelings people expect you to have – being grateful you've got one, knowing you can conceive, counting your blessings – and the feelings you experience every day – sadness, frustration, anger and guilt – can become unbearable. As with everything else in fertility treatment, no one can wave a magic wand and make it all right, but telling someone how you feel may make you feel less alone.

10

The Emotional Journey: Secrecy and Support

B eing told that you may never have children, or being told that your only hope of having children is with medical intervention, is a crisis – often a crisis that couples keep to themselves. Janice says,

'We got married expecting to have a family, and it took us ten years to have Lily. I knew people who had had trouble, but I never thought it would happen to me.'

That sense of surprise is widespread. Many of us imagine the children we might have one day, and they can come to seem real. Gail feels 'cheated' because of her miscarriage.

'We so nearly had a child – that's what seems so unfair.'

Equally widespread is the certainty that, once you do begin treatment, all your problems will be solved. Mira recalls,

'I assumed that I'd be able to get pregnant as soon as I came off the pill, and it didn't happen. Then I assumed that once I started on Clomid, I'd get pregnant, and it didn't happen. Then I assumed that once we started IVF treatment I'd get pregnant, and it didn't happen. I'm only just now beginning to face up to the fact that it may never happen at all.'

Jana found that her doubts and worries surfaced in dreams, rather than consciously.

'When we were first trying, I had a series of nightmares in which I'd got a baby, but it wasn't the right one, and I went down to the river and put it in a basket and watched it float away. In the mornings I'd wake crying, knowing I'd given up my only chance to have a baby.'

GUILT AND FAILURE

For some women, the experience of infertility stirs up complicated and ambiguous emotions that they find it hard to share, as it did for Karen.

'I had an abortion when I was 19. Now that I'm 34, I've spent ten years trying to get pregnant without success. No one ever makes the wrong choice in life. We always make the best choice as it seems to us at the time. I can't change the choice I made, but I'm left with a sense of profound sadness and regret.'

Some women are able to put the past behind them and concentrate on finding a solution to the problems of the present, but it's not always so simple. Carmel feels guilt at a previous termination even more strongly:

'It's hard not to see what's happening to me now as punishment for what I did then. What's worse is, of course, that there may be a connection. If there was an infection, or scar tissue. . . . I'm only able to think that I brought this on myself.'

Certainly, when treatment first begins, everyone's hopes are raised. Callie says,

'Early on, I could feel hopeful quite easily. I thought then that medical science had an answer for everything. Now I know how much they still

don't know about the seemingly simple task of getting pregnant. I become increasingly desperate and despondent.'

So many times, when I was talking to women, the past few years of their lives seemed to be summed up in their treatments: 'I've had three IVFs, two miscarriages, four IUIs, one ICSI . . .', or their struggle to find out what was wrong: 'By then we were on our fourth doctor. . . .' It took 'five or six years' for doctors to find out that Maria wasn't ovulating, 'and only then did I get on to the real treatment that I needed.'

The emotional impact on anyone undertaking prolonged treatment for infertility cannot be overestimated. Many counsellors say that coping with infertility is like coping with bereavement: couples go through many of the same emotions – shock, anger, denial . . . But, as Maria points out,

'With infertility you have to cope with that bereavement and the sense of failure that it brings every single month.'

The constant 'failure' as month after month goes by can strike deep at a woman's sense of self. Sophie says,

'I felt so useless, I used to think to myself, 16-year-olds do this. Why can't I?'

Richard found it very difficult to know what to say to Rosemary, either in the early days when another month went by and it was clear they hadn't conceived again, and also later, when they were undergoing treatments which failed.

'She was the one bearing the weight of it all. She had to watch for signs of ovulation, wonder whether she was pregnant . . . As she put it, all I had to do was have sex and wait and see what happened. She was living with it much more closely than I was. I was also more optimistic. Part of me just wondered when this would all stop so life could get back to normal.'

It can be especially difficult if your own work brings you into contact with children. Ellen, who is a social worker, finds that most days she comes into contact

'with families who can't cope with their children, who are having problems with their children, and now and again mothers who are pregnant who don't want any more children. There is nothing I can say sometimes when they tell me they wish they'd never had children in the first place. What can I possibly say to them?'

Roseanne found her feelings becoming more negative:

'I told myself that this was God's plan for me. This helped me get over some of the difficult times, because I thought I was learning some very hard lessons and that I would grow and come out of the experience a stronger human being and a better parent because of it. But now I wonder if God's simply got my plan mixed up with someone else's. I don't see anything positive any more in this, just pain.'

Callie also has

'a hard time battling against being depressed and sad all the time . . . I try not to let it take all the joy out of my life, but there are days when it feels like it has.'

Like many people, Eilish sometimes has doubts about going on:

'Every treatment that fails makes you feel more of a failure than ever. Not only that, it makes you think that there must be something really wrong with you if you can't conceive after all this high-tech help.'

But how hard it is not to go on. Gilli says,

'The struggle takes you over. I sometimes stop and wonder who I might have been if I hadn't had this problem and had been allowed to have a normal life.'

Lena often has doubt about continuing treatment:

'Some days, I really wonder what we are doing to ourselves, our marriage, the rest of our family . . . Why do we feel so compelled to have children when, if advanced technologies didn't exist, we would have no hope of conceiving?'

THE IMPACT ON YOUR RELATIONSHIP

So why do we feel so compelled to go on? Christine, whose partner Brian already has two children from his first marriage, thinks she has an answer to that question.

'I think in the end it comes down to biological instinct. And instincts are very strong. It's biologically natural for us to feel this way. Every creature on this earth has reproduction as its main goal. I can understand why I feel the way I do, but Brian can't because he's already fulfilled that goal.'

Christine is finding that Brian cannot understand the intensity of her feelings and, although they are going through IVF treatment together, she feels that she has been the one to drive the process along. Sara felt something of that too:

'I always thought that David would have accepted childlessness much more easily than me, and I think that was because he didn't have a problem. Because it was my problem, I felt like I had to put it right.'

Deirdre, on the other hand, is worried that her probable inability to have children, because of severe endometriosis, will mean the end of her marriage.

'I don't know if our relationship can survive this. When we got married it was with the idea that the time was now right to start a family of our own. Where does that leave us if that isn't going to happen?'

Liz too feels under pressure:

'Steve's been very supportive, done every test that's needed to be done, come along with me to my treatments . . . It's hard knowing that the problem lies with just me, not him. We were at a wedding a few weeks ago and there were so many children there, and one of my cousins said how good he was with the kids . . . He'd make a good dad – that's why it's so hard for us to deal with this. We go through different phases: some days I think we should make a definite decision to adopt, other days I don't want to because I want Steve to have the chance to have a baby of his own. I want to have a baby who looks like him. There's just no clear direction.'

This uncertainty means living in a permanent 'crisis' state. Janice says,

'It can take you over, the idea of a baby. Your whole world becomes unreal sometimes. Even hours can seem like forever when you're feeling low, and the years of treatment can feel like centuries. The burden on a couple is enormous. It will bring you together or pull you apart.'

Certainly, if you are both committed to the treatment it can make life easier. Gilli, aware of her partner Adam's ambivalence when treatment began, was also aware of her own 'desperate desire' to have a baby:

'I tried to take as much of the stress of treatment as I could – tablets, injections, endless scans and hospital visits – and I withdrew from Adam because of this. We became more distant and irritable with each other just when we needed more support than ever.'

DISCLOSURE

Although our society is becoming more accepting of infertility, and there is more freedom to make individual choices, needing medical help to conceive is a fact that many couples are reluctant to share, especially while they're undergoing treatment. Karen resents the way people ask questions:

'First there's "How long have you been married?" then there's "Do you have any children?" And if we say no, there's "How long are you going to wait before you start a family?" It's none of their business. I don't want our problems and decisions to be the topic of everyone's small talk.'

Perhaps not everyone will take the need to keep things to themselves as far as Sara and David did. Sara, who spent 14 years trying to conceive, says,

'We kept it very quiet. I told my best friend, but she's in Australia. We didn't tell anybody about the tests or the treatment until Thomas was born. If things had gone wrong, we couldn't have coped if people had known. And when we did find out we were expecting, we still didn't tell anyone. I wasn't working, so there were no work colleagues to tell. For a start, we found it very hard to believe in the pregnancy ourselves. So when he did arrive it was a surprise all round, not least because he came five weeks early. The neighbours wondered where we'd got this baby from. Quite a few people thought we'd adopted. But funnily enough, no one has ever asked us why we kept it to ourselves. It's as if they know.'

Keeping your situation secret has its price. Marion says,

'It was such an effort sometimes not to lash out at people for being insensitive, although I hadn't given them any reason to think that there was something I might be sensitive to.'

Amanda too has kept her feelings to herself:

'I know there is a general view at work that I'm being selfish, that I don't want to disrupt my career, sacrifice my salary. I know that's what people think of me. But how can I tell them what I'm really going through?'

Couples without children may also find themselves being envied. Carol says,

'People say how lucky we are that we could have these wonderful holidays and things. But we want a child to have those holidays with.'

One reason many couples decide not to share what's happening to them is the difficulty of dealing with other people's opinions. When Matt told colleagues at work that he and his partner were having IVF treatment, he found very little support.

'People would say, "Why don't you adopt?", as if it was the answer to all the world's problems. They implied that we were selfish to want a child when there were already so many unloved children in the world, as if we could just go out and adopt one of them.'

Tanya met a similar reaction:

'People say to me, "Why don't you just adopt?", but this implies that adoption is easy, and even if it was, it's not something you "just" do.'

Alison only realised how much she and Peter, who has a spinal injury, had kept things to themselves when, while having IVF treatment, she met someone she used to be at school with.

'She had such a distinctive voice and I heard her across the waiting room . . . Luckily, we weren't still in touch and didn't still have mutual

contacts, so I knew she wasn't going to spread the word back, and neither was I, but it made me think about how little we had told anyone. We hadn't even told my mother-in-law that we were having treatment. I don't know how she thinks we ever conceived Christopher. It wasn't that we were keeping the treatment secret, just that we didn't want to have to explain things to people all of the time. The more people you tell, the more expectations are raised, and we didn't want to raise our hopes too high.'

For all these reasons, couples keep quiet, but Gilli found the isolation hard to bear.

'The doctors can be nice, but they didn't seem to understand or cope particularly well when I broke down in tears. So I had to hold myself together for others as well as for myself, which made me withdraw further into myself and become more isolated.'

Isolation, at a time of your life when you need more support than ever, is an added burden, but finding someone you can talk to, to help ease that burden, is not an easy task. Amanda is dismissive:

'Of course we haven't told many people. Even the few people we have told can't understand what we're going through. How can they? They're all parents.'

Signs that you need more support
- when you find yourself crying for no reason
- when you can't tell your partner how you really feel
- when you feel you have no one to talk to
- when you feel nobody understands

FINDING SUPPORT

Perhaps the most obvious place to turn is to your partner. Some couples find that the experience of infertility brings them closer together, but it is very rare for any couple to come through the experience without mild disagreements, heated arguments and blazing rows. All your usual ways of supporting each other may have dissipated over the weeks, months or years of waiting. Sex has probably become a weary chore, undertaken when the date is right, even if your libido has evaporated. Physically intrusive tests and investigations may mean that you can never think quite the same way again about the most intimate aspects of your bodies. But if you can't talk to your partner about how you feel, who can you turn to?

Friends

Although friends may be a natural place to turn, what if they are having babies left, right and centre? Roseanne says,

'Every one – and I really mean every single one – of my friends has children now.'

When friends and relatives are having babies of their own, this can prove a real crisis point. Sara remembers,

'My friend phoned me one Christmas Eve to tell me she'd just found out she was pregnant. I was very pleased for her – of course I was – but you can be pleased while still feeling your own distress.'

Deanne finally told her best friend what she was going through when that friend had a baby and asked her to be godmother.

'I was very happy for her when she and her husband conceived – at first go, I think – but that hasn't stopped me crying nearly every time I see

my godson. When things go right for others, it's just a huge reminder that things aren't going right for you, and it hurts. Sometimes that has to spill out.'

Ellen also found that the truth 'spilled out' one day when she lost her temper with her sister:

'She was always going on to me about how having a baby was such hard work and so tiring and she never got any sleep . . . and then she tells me that she's having a second one. I didn't see why she should be, when all she had ever done to me was complain, and I shouted that if she found she couldn't have children then she'd have something to complain about.'

Sunita also finds it hard to take when

'Even people who have struggled to have children complain about them. How easily they forget how lucky they are. And those who have never needed treatment to have children, they just don't know how lucky they are.'

Lena, too, finds her temper fraying at times:

'When I told my friend that we were trying, she said, "Oh, I know what it's like. We had to wait, too." She took three months to conceive.'

Family

Relatives can sometimes be supportive, but what if your parents make heavy hints about how long you're making them wait to become grandparents? And what if your sister is making the most of your child-free status by using you as a twice-a-week babysitter for her brood of three? She may delight more in telling you about the downside of parenting than in summoning up the energy to understand your feelings.

Mira admits,

'My family don't know what to say to me or how to say it. They get awkward when they tell me about christenings coming up, or one of my cousins getting married because she found she was expecting. Most of the time we don't say anything if we can help it.'

Dealing with your family can be difficult if you are expected to turn up to celebrations where babies and children will be present, and there are days when you just don't feel you can deal with this. Jayne says,

'Christmas was always a difficult time. One year my husband's brother and wife came over from America and we were expected to spend Christmas with them. They had two babies. My period was due on Christmas Day. I had to do a pregnancy test in the morning and if it failed – which it did – sit and enjoy a wonderful day with them. I said I couldn't go. I would have hated to have ruined their Christmas. I stayed away but insisted my husband go for the morning. He came back in tears. He felt very envious of their joy and seeing the children open their presents . . .'

Karen told her family and wishes she hadn't.

'They just try to help with their pearls of wisdom, which only make me feel worse. They're always saying things like, "You've got plenty of time yet, don't worry about it . . ." They don't understand.'

Work colleagues

Jana found that her work colleagues jumped to conclusions:

'I was seen as someone very dependable. Even when other women were taking maternity leave, it was like they could always rely on me because I wasn't going to do anything like that in the middle of a

project. It felt very hurtful, but it was true. I could be relied upon. That was what was so sad.'

That's one drawback of keeping things to yourself. But what if you are honest? You may find that work colleagues write off your career prospects because you may disappear to Planet Motherhood at any moment. Also, what are you going to say when you need time off work for tests and treatments? If you don't tell anyone, you'll come under even more stress as you have to invent reasons for your absences.

Support organisations

Many women feel that in their immediate circle of friends and family there is no one who quite understands what they're going through. Marion says:

'No one in my life can understand the heartbreak I feel, because for them it's all come very easily.'

This is where organisations which can offer support really come into their own, because through them you will find people in a similar position to your own and willing to talk openly about their own problems in a way that will make you feel less alone with yours.

Sara found the telephone helpline of the self-help organisation CHILD a useful source of support. In addition, she always made sure she got the information she needed when making decisions.

'I was always phoning the HFEA and asking them about success rates, and this mixture of up-to-date and reliable information together with understanding and support is something the national organisations are particularly well equipped to do.'

However, you do have to pay to join some organisations, and Gail couldn't afford it:

'I know it's not a lot, but we looked into joining at a time when we were having to pay for our first IUI – which was £550 – and we just couldn't.'

Through CHILD, Gilli met two other women who lived near her and were going through IVF:

'Although our circumstances were different, it was such a help to talk to someone who really knew what you were talking about, and such a relief to know that we weren't alone. Outside of this, I found it hard to share what I really felt. Unless you've been there, how can you understand the despair and the unfairness of it all?'

Yet Hannah, who has been trying for two years ('ever since my thirtieth birthday'), doesn't see any value for her in support groups.

'I don't want to join a group of other childless women. I don't like to think of myself that way, and to join a group would be to sign up for membership of something I never want to be.'

Carol went to several meetings of the patient support group at the clinic where she was having treatment.

'Some days I came out of it feeling really good. I was encouraged by all the success stories that we heard and made me think we were in with a good chance. Other days I'd come out with a feeling that nothing was ever going to go right for us. If I met someone who'd just got a positive result, I'd get irritated, thinking that they were using up all the good chances. There were always going to be people in that support group who weren't successful, and if it wasn't them, it was more likely to be me. Even hearing myself say this, I know how insane it sounds, but statistically, of course, I'm right.'

Many hospitals and treatment centres have patient support groups, which often meet monthly and aim to provide a safe, friendly environment where people can share their fears, hopes and emotional turmoil. If you can't face going to a group, many clinics can put you in touch with other patients who have volunteered their names for one-to-one contact and support.

Counselling

If you are undertaking IVF or any treatment involving donor gametes, your treatment centre must offer you counselling, though not all couples take advantage of this. Sara, when she was considering IVF with donated eggs, found it valuable:

'The counsellor did raise quite a few things that we needed to think through. It's important, if you have any doubts at all about your treatment, to talk them through first.'

Jenny, who is a counsellor herself, found that it offered her and her partner, Greg, a small, private time and space to air worries that had been troubling them with the 'safety' of a third party in the room.

'There were things I found difficult to say, and it was sometimes easier to say them to someone who wasn't going to leap to conclusions, or rush to judge me, than to say them directly to Greg. Especially when I was confused about whether we should go on. We'd invested so much time, money and hope in IVF working that I knew Greg didn't want to face the possibility that it might not work. But after two cycles had ended in failure, I felt it was important that we start to look at a future where we stopped treatment.'

Anne had counselling but didn't find it helpful at the time:

'I thought that the only solution I needed to my "problems" was getting pregnant, not talking about how I felt about not getting pregnant.

Anyway, I could only cope with all the invasive treatments by shutting away my feelings – anger, sadness, confusion.'

Colleen, too, found it difficult at first to feel that talking with a counsellor was helping:

'I cried the whole time, and she told me I was depressed about something I couldn't just make happen. Well, I knew all that. But gradually, over a few sessions, we talked about this depression, and I realised it wasn't just depression – it was grief. I was grieving. And that made me feel better on the days when I had to let my feelings out and have a cry. She made me feel that crying was one way of keeping strong, by letting out the feelings every so often. I recognised that I could have bad days but I would still have the strength to keep going.'

Letting feelings out can be an important part of counselling. If you feel very angry all the time, this can get bottled up and you are likely to find yourself hitting out at your partner or some other unsuspecting person. Jenny says,

'Thinking I might never have children made me feel desperate, absolutely desperate. If I hadn't had someone I could talk to, to express just how shredded I felt by the idea that I might never ever be pregnant in my whole life, I'd have gone insane.'

Deirdre found that counselling helped when she was feeling very low and contemplating giving up treatment completely.

'What got to me was hearing other people's happy stories at our support group all the time. They'd all end with the phrase "Miracles do happen!" And I was convinced, deep down, that they weren't going to happen to me. Talking those feelings through really helped.'

Talking with a counsellor is not a sign that you can't cope. You've
never had to face a situation like this before, so it's no wonder you
find it hard to pin down exactly what you feel – and you may well
need a chance to talk it all through before you know exactly what
your feelings are. Knowing that counselling is confidential, that you
won't be told to buck your ideas up or to be grateful for all the
wonderful things in life you've already got, or that the person
you're talking to won't immediately run to the consultant in charge
of your treatment and tell him that under no circumstances must
you be allowed to be a parent because you're so unstable, can
provide you with the safety valve you need.

Even when things are apparently going well – your pregnancy
test has come back positive, say – you might want to talk to
someone. How can you tell the friend you've come to rely on
that you're pregnant, when her own cycle has just ended in
failure? Who are you going to tell that being pregnant, after all
this time, fills you with fear and dread rather than happiness? It's
a fact that some women, sometimes after years of intense treatment, have a termination when they find out that they're
pregnant, especially if they have been focusing on the idea of
pregnancy all the time and then don't feel ready to have a child.
Sara talked these things through with her counsellor, who
reassured her that having doubts about being pregnant with
donated eggs was not unusual.

*'She said that people often have doubts about the pregnancy anyway,
and if they've used donated sperm or eggs, they put their feelings of
unease down to the donation. But it generally goes deeper than that – a
feeling that they've made a mistake going through with treatment at
all.'*

Another thing that Sara found reassuring to hear from her counsellor was the fact that any lingering doubts usually disperse
immediately the baby is born:

'She said she'd never met a woman who had a problem afterwards. It's in the initial stages of pregnancy that the doubts are strong, and if you can get past that you'll be okay.'

Ilona admits,

'I'd thought that counselling was going to be absolutely useless, I had these visions of lying on a couch and wittering on about wanting a baby. But when I got there, I felt like I was sorting things out for myself. It was the one thing that made me feel in control when everything else was out of my control.'

Internet resources

A great deal of health information, some of it more reliable than the rest, is available on the Internet. On web sites set up by large organisations you can find the results of studies published in medical journals, where facts are backed up with clinical trial evidence. You can also find informal groups which offer much in the way of emotional support and encouragement – but be wary of opinions put forward as established fact.

Sometimes you can find out facts which are very helpful, and the answers to questions you may not have thought to ask when you were with your consultant. Sharon, who was told she had a 'tilted uterus' left after her appointment and only later thought of the questions she wanted to ask.

'Would it make it more difficult for me to get pregnant? Would it lead to a higher risk of miscarriage? Did anything need to be done about it? Could anything be done about it? Given that my cervix wasn't in the normal place, should we be having sex in different positions if we wanted to get pregnant? Well, sometimes you don't want to ask your consultant questions like that, and sometimes you're afraid to ask the most basic questions because everyone seems to assume you know all about it. I was able to do some research that night and get most of my

questions answered from a reputable medical library, which was much better than lying awake worrying about it.'

The most important thing to remember is that no one can give you patient-specific advice online. Only your own GP or consultant knows your full case history and circumstances, has carried out any tests, and has made decisions about your treatment in the light of what he or she knows about you as a particular couple. You can get general information which can be extremely valuable, but it cannot replace the specific advice your own doctor will be able to provide.

The causes and treatments of infertility are constantly being studied, and a great deal of research is currently being done into immune factor infertility, for example, so you may read of amazing new treatments or drug regimes online, but you cannot assume that they will necessarily be appropriate for you. A new approach may still be part of a clinical trial, and may pose risks to you which on balance your doctor feels must rule the treatment out.

However, with these warnings in place, the more information you have about your situation, your condition, the treatments open to you and the avenues you could pursue, the better understanding you will have of the choices available to you – an understanding which will help you get more out of your meetings with your doctor. Danny Tucker, a Specialist Registrar in Obstetrics and Gynaecology at Jessop Hospital for Women, Sheffield, maintains the Pregnancy and Women's Health Information web site pages for this very reason.

'I believe that people, in the UK particularly, don't know enough about their health problems or understand properly the decisions they are asked to make. Things are improving and most hospitals have information sheets now on conditions, procedures and operations, but there is still a way to go. I truly believe that an informed patient gets more from the health service.'

There is a list of web sites which can offer you information on p. 288.

Newsgroups

One useful innovation in the world of information-exchange has been the development of worldwide support and information groups (Usenet) which you can access via the Internet. There are over twenty-five thousand newsgroups discussing every subject under the sun, but out of this encyclopaedia of interests you will find newsgroups that discuss topics relevant to couples in the infertility maze. Newsgroups work a bit like bulletin boards: any-one can post a message on the board to share information, or post a question for others to answer, and you can then respond to or comment on these messages or post one of your own. Some newsgroups are 'moderated', which means that articles must be sent to a moderator for approval before appearing in the news-group, but most are unmoderated. Some groups are very busy, while others only have a couple of messages posted per week.

Many groups have an introductory message which is posted at intervals, often called the FAQ (Frequently Asked Questions); this describes the content and purpose of the newsgroup. Until you're familiar with a newsgroup you cannot have a feeling for the subjects up for discussion, the rules of politeness or whether someone's just asked a question you want to ask. . . . So follow the group for a while and, when you feel you've got to know it, join in if you want.

Simone has been trying to conceive for a year and confesses to being a 'newbie' to newsgroups.

'But I've found the postings very helpful, not so much in terms of information, but because it helps to know that there are so many people out there going through the same spectrum of emotions as we are. We're always told we're not alone with our infertility, but it feels like it.'

For some couples, newsgroups prove a useful source of emotional support because you can:

- find out how other people are feeling who are going through situations similar to your own
- listen in to discussions without anyone knowing you're there
- choose to participate only if you wish
- participate anonymously if you wish

While you can never base your choices about what treatments and options would be right for you entirely on the basis of other people's experiences, sharing those experiences can provide you with support at a vulnerable time. There is a list of newsgroups active at the time of writing on p. 296.

Mailing lists

There are several open mailing lists which have been formed to discuss topics related to infertility. Gail currently subscribes to the e-mail support group ONNA – as in, Oh No, Not (my period) Again – and has found it 'a ray of sunshine'. She feels that

'It's a two-way thing. You've got to support other people because you know what they're going through. At one point I unsubscribed when our treatment failed, because I couldn't carry on supporting other people. Then I needed support again, so I resubscribed. I've met a lot of people through the group – some I e-mail a couple of times a week.'

Sometimes you will need support at specific times, even though the rest of the time you are happy to go it alone. Maggie says,

'Doing IVF is emotionally and physically intense. If you can get together with other people who are going through it at about the same time as

you are, it can make all the difference. I was part of an e-mail support group for January IVFers, and it was a lifeline in terms of information and emotional support.'

Deborah found the instant support she received at specific times in her treatments very valuable.

'I got so many messages of goodwill when we were going through our IUIs that it really made me feel we weren't going through the journey alone. I was able to wake up and face each new day knowing there were people out there with me.'

Gail, too, enjoyed the sense of community.

'There were all these women, keeping each other updated on their treatments and progress and whether their period had started or not, and what their ultrasound had felt like . . . Sometimes when someone went away from the list for a while, perhaps because they were in hospital for treatment, you were on tenterhooks waiting for them to come back and tell you the results.'

On the other hand, as with any support group, sometimes the stories of others can be too much to bear. Are they telling your their story from the heady heights of a successful treatment, or the jaundiced viewpoint of a recently unsuccessful one? Often it seems as if others are making headway with their treatments, even if it's just to report that such-and-such a test was done, while you're being left behind, especially if you're on a waiting list whose summit never seems to get any nearer. At least mailing lists offer you the chance to drop in and a listen for a while, or stay away for a while, in a manner that can suit your emotional needs and without having to explain your decisions to anyone else. So if you want to ask others who have been there about your strange temperature charts for this month, or let everyone know you've just had trouble coping at a family wedding, then mailing lists will have a lot to offer you, in terms not just of information but also of support. If your fellow listees know you are going for your embryo transfer, for example, you will receive a lot of individual messages of goodwill, and that in itself can make you feel less alone.

Further information about some of the mailing lists currently running can be found on p. 300.

11

When Treatment Results in a Pregnancy

Donna says,

'I'd begun to think it would never happen to me. We'd been trying for about three and a half years altogether, and after our second IVF cycle I got a positive pregnancy test. I thought I was dreaming. In fact I was sure I was dreaming and would wake up soon. I walked around most of the day in a daze, hardly able to think straight. I was more hesitant than happy.'

Sally mentions the same word, 'hesitant', when describing how she felt when the test turned positive.

'I was so excited but so hesitant. It seems so unfair for all of us who've waited so long for that moment that we can't just let ourselves enjoy it because we can never feel totally sure. I think we know more than anyone what a long way we've still got to go.'

Leona remembers seeing two sacs on her first ultrasound and reacted only with 'guarded optimism'.

'I knew how early it was, and I'd had too many disappointments in the past to get really excited. It's awful that the experience of infertility makes you damp down your emotions like that.'

Alison, too, kept her emotions in check for quite a while after her positive pregnancy test.

'I refused to let myself think it was going to happen for about the first three months, because I was aware of the high rate of ectopics that can follow treatment. So although we were happy, there were all these other worries, too.'

Recognising an ectopic

It's essential that an ectopic pregnancy is recognised as soon as possible because the internal bleeding it causes can be life-threatening. The first signs can be abdominal pain, vaginal bleeding or sometimes a 'referred' pain in your shoulder, caused by a build-up of blood which is increasing the pressure in your abdomen. The best ways of identifying an ectopic are through early scans, and checking the levels of hCG in the woman's bloodstream. If you have an ectopic pregnancy, you may well continue to feel pregnant, or you may find that your early pregnancy symptoms fade because the embryo has already perished.

Sara couldn't really take in the fact that she was pregnant until about 20 weeks. Peter found that his sense of worry lasted even longer:

'It persisted for about six months. Only when we'd got to the stage where the baby would be okay anyway did it start to fade.'

Many women have a sense of worry and uncertainty in the early weeks of pregnancy, but these feelings seem to be highlighted for couples who have waited a long time for a baby, perhaps because they have learned the value of caution. And there does need to be caution along with the hope and delight. A 'clinical pregnancy' (defined as one where the presence of a foetal heart has been detected at about seven weeks of gestation) doesn't always lead to a live birth. IVF parents have a higher than normal risk (2 per cent) of an ectopic pregnancy,[8] or there may be a distressing miscarriage.

However, the miscarriage rate for viable IVF pregnancies (about 8 per cent) doesn't seem to be significantly higher than for spontaneous pregnancies.

No matter how much reassurance you get from medical staff, and no matter how closely you are monitored, many couples who have conceived as a result of assisted conception will spend a significant percentage of their pregnancy worrying about the outcome. Majella thought her pregnancy was going to feel like floating along on a cloud:

'I expected to feel over the moon the whole time. I was certainly very happy, but it seemed like every magazine or newsletter I picked up was packed with stories of babies who needed special care.'

Jenny, who experienced some spotting in the early weeks, felt as if

'the black cloud of our bad luck which had been hanging over us through all the years when we were having treatment was still hanging over us, threatening to rain. It didn't seem fair that I couldn't participate in the pregnancy as much as other mothers at my antenatal clinic seemed to. I couldn't let myself trust it would all be okay.'

In addition, pregnancy after assisted conception can bring its own unique problems. Ruth had a positive pregnancy test after her second attempt at IVF, when she had three embryos transferred, but started to bleed shortly afterwards.

'I phoned the clinic in a lather and they told me to lie down and rest, and reassured me that it might be just one of the implanted embryos coming away. Luckily it was, and the pregnancy continued without any more trouble.'

Some women do experience slight cramping around the time of implantation – twinges that mightn't even be noticed in a normal pregnancy, but which can cause extreme worry when you are hyper-alert to what may be happening inside you. Slight spotting may happen and cause you untold concern. Angela found that for the first few days after her pregnancy test came back positive she felt as if she were 'walking on glass':

'I was afraid to sneeze, I was afraid to cough. If I could have padded my stomach all around with cotton wool, I would have.'

As with any pregnancy, your body is going through major changes, and as it adjusts the stress can be overwhelming. Kathleen was very aware of pains in her right side after her first pregnancy test had come back positive.

'I was convinced I had an ectopic, absolutely convinced. I didn't really let go of this fear until I had an ultrasound and saw for myself that everything was where it should be. And then, of course, the pains started fading away.'

It's not unknown for couples to experience some ambivalence when the pregnancy test finally turns positive. Deirdre says,

'I was shocked, My first thought was, "Am I really ready for this?" We'd had a big struggle and we'd been battling and battling, and it was hard to accept that the battle was now over. We'd tried so hard to achieve this, and now it was here and I felt guilty that I wasn't overwhelmed with pleasure. It seemed like I was never going to leave guilt behind.'

Liam was more prepared for his feelings:

'I knew from talking to other fathers that that there was often some ambivalence when they first found out a baby was on the way. Because there is ambivalence. Not only do you start to worry how your partner will cope physically and whether the baby will be okay, but about money and . . . about everything.'

Perhaps understandably, babies born as a result of IVF have been studied closely for many years to check how they develop into children. All the evidence suggests that their risk of being born with an abnormality is no more than that for children conceived naturally.

MORE THAN YOU BARGAINED FOR?

Assisted conception does, however, increase the possibility of a multiple pregnancy, particularly if the maximum three embryos are transferred during IVF. There are rare occurrences of pregnancies of six, seven or more, which usually happen after superovulation treatment. Nowadays safeguards are built into the process to avoid this, and you will be advised not to have intercourse or AI on a cycle where ultrasound monitoring shows an unusually large number of developing follicles.

Multiple outcomes

Out of 6721 clinical pregnancies following IVF or frozen embryo transfer: reported to the HFEA for their *Sixth Annual Report:*

- 4782 were singletons
- 1678 were twins
- 255 were triplets
- 6 were quads

Not all clinical pregnancies result in a live birth, but these figures show that the possibility of a multiple birth cannot be discounted. Around 25 per cent of couples who have had IVF treatment will have twins (compared to one in 90 of the rest of the population), and just under 5 per cent will have triplets (compared to one in 9000).

Whilst many couples who want a baby are quite happy to risk having twins or triplets, there are very few who would choose to start their family with triplets. Even those who are initially delighted at the prospect may find that doubts creep in, especially as the pregnancy progresses and they begin to wonder how they will cope.

If you are carrying more than one baby, you will usually be told this news at an early ultrasound scan. Some parents will be thrilled. Others will have concerns about practical and financial considerations after the babies arrive, and yet others will worry throughout the pregnancy about problems in labour and the health of the babies.

The average length of a twin pregnancy is around 37 weeks, compared to 40 weeks for a single child. Triplets and quads also tend to arrive earlier, so if you do have a multiple pregnancy your babies run a high risk of being born prematurely (although many twins are just as healthy and heavy at birth as singletons). Many multiples are born without serious problems, but most triplets and many twins will need to be looked after in a special care baby unit, sometimes for several weeks. The stillbirth and neonatal death rate for triplets conceived through IVF is much greater than for singletons,[9] and if very premature babies do survive, they have a higher risk of mental and physical disabilities.

All of these facts (which are not set down here purely to alarm you, but to help you assess the risks and choices you may have to face in the future) can make a multiple pregnancy a worrying time. If you find out you are carrying more than one baby, you will need extra support from your partner and from family and friends. Support groups such as TAMBA (Twins and Multiple Births Association; see p. 286) can also offer information and advice to help you through your pregnancy and prepare you for labour. As Majella says, when she found that she was carrying three babies,

'I'd spent so many years not having any children, then I thought I might have the hope of one – and now suddenly I found I was going to

have three all at once. That's quite a mental step for anyone to have to take.'

Early twins

Since ultrasound scanning has become a routine procedure in early pregnancy, it's now known that many mothers who conceive twins (whether through assisted conception techniques or not) go on to give birth to a single baby. At one time, no one would ever have known of the second baby's existence. For parents, the complex emotions of grief for the 'lost' baby can be caught up with a sense of thankfulness but concern for the survivor.

Leona had a twin implantation but gave birth to just one baby:

'I saw two sacs on the ultrasound the first time, and we'd sort of expected this as our first pregnancy test was very, very, very positive – the hCG was very high. But we went on to have Daisy. It helped that I was told that up to one in five conceptions is initially a twin conception naturally, so it felt like something natural.'

Monica found that it affected her more deeply:

'At my second ultrasound we found that one of the embryos was developing well, and we even saw a tiny flicker which we were told was the heartbeat. But the other embryo had started shrinking. The doctor said it might still develop, but was probably a vanishing twin and would disintegrate and be reabsorbed. I felt guilty for feeling so sad about this. I knew that one baby was still okay, and I should count myself lucky because so many people go through several IVFs and are never successful at all . . . But it left me feeling that I still couldn't trust the rest of the pregnancy to be okay. I was always worrying and wondering.'

MIRACLE PREGNANCY

The extent to which infertility clinics remain involved with a couple after treatment will vary, although the clinic will want to know the outcome of your treatment for its own records. Often, once pregnancy is established, patients return to the care of their own GPs or local hospitals.

There's no reason why, once it's safely established, a pregnancy after infertility treatment shouldn't proceed just as any other pregnancy would, although many parents feel that it seems to last longer because it's usually diagnosed earlier. Even if you're carrying twins or triplets, you may not feel any physical difference apart from being larger and more uncomfortable at an earlier stage. For Gilli, this very normality was a problem:

'You make the transition from infertility treatment to antenatal care very quickly, and in the antenatal clinic you're just one of the crowd again. I didn't feel like one of the crowd. I wanted a label saying "Miracle baby" pasted at the top of my notes.'

Also, as Monica found, many parents miss the support of their consultants or patient support groups.

'I used to rely a lot on the support of people who were going through infertility treatment with us, and with the positive pregnancy test that support seemed suddenly withdrawn.'

Sara, on the other hand, found her pregnancy 'absolutely wonderful' in every way.

'Once we knew I had a viable pregnancy, I was back to normal – no longer down and very depressed all the time. The contrast was staggering. I had some sickness early on, but we took that as only a positive sign. I was so full of energy – it was like a weight had been

removed. David said that he'd forgotten how full of energy I always used to be.'

Of course, you can also feel the usual side-effects of pregnancy: the high levels of hCG that are circulating in your body, especially in the first trimester, can make you nauseous, tired and extremely emotional. Or positively euphoric and radiant.

PROGESTERONE SUPPLEMENTS

When the pregnancy was conceived by IVF, the usual support mechanisms from the corpus luteum (which develops in the follicle after ovulation) have not developed, and progesterone must be given to sustain the pregnancy. Whether you are given it through injections, suppositories or micronised oral tablets will be up to your consultant. All are equally effective, but they may have to juggle the doses to get the right amount into your bloodstream because people absorb substances to different degrees.

Because of recurrent miscarriages after previous IVF treatments, Sara was on a double dose of progesterone for the first 16 weeks of her pregnancy. She found her injections very unpleasant.

'We'd done three cycles almost back to back, January, April and July, so I still hadn't recovered in any of my injection sites and the injections in my legs were excruciatingly painful. But I would do it all again.'

Alison found her injections so painful that she stopped having them at 12 weeks.

'I said I just couldn't stand it any more, and if it wasn't meant to be by now then it wasn't meant to be.'

ANTENATAL TESTS

Babies conceived through assisted conception can still be at risk of chromosomal and congenital abnormalities in the way that any other baby would be, although there's no increased risk. You may therefore be faced with another barrage of choices and worries through early pregnancy if you're offered antenatal scans and tests. The tests you're offered will vary according to your hospital, your health authority and your age. The more information you have about these tests, the more you'll understand what risks and choices you have, and what possible consequences you face which-ever way you decide. Sometimes you have to be persistent in asking for more information. Midwives are usually happy to talk to you about the tests and any worries you may have, and the hospital doctor and your own GP can give you further information if you need it. Some parents find it very helpful to talk to a counsellor, too, either before having any tests or when thinking through some difficult decisions.

Thinking about tests

You might find it helpful to talk through questions such as these with hospital staff or a counsellor:

- is this a test we want?
- is there a risk to the baby?
- who can help us deal with our anxieties?
- what will we do if the tests show the baby is at risk of chromosomal abnormality?

Sara and David decided that they were not going to have any invasive tests, but decided to have the nuchal scan as they were having ultrasound scans anyway. In this test, which uses ultra-sound, the nuchal fold at the back of the baby's neck is measured. A wider than usual fold can indicate an increased risk of Down's syndrome. Sara says,

'We had this for reassurance, but I honestly don't know how we would have felt if the results had come back showing a big risk, because we'd already decided that we wouldn't terminate.'

Leona was initially reluctant to have any tests:

'I was offered the triple test [a blood test offered in early pregnancy to help assess the risk of having a baby with Down's syndrome or neural tube detects such as spina bifida] and felt pressured into having it because of my age – I was 38. I only went ahead with it because I never for a moment believed there would be anything wrong with the baby. And don't forget, at this point I still hadn't really taken in that I was pregnant, so in a way I felt that it was all theoretical and I think that's why we finally went ahead.'

The results of the triple test are expressed in terms of risk, whether parents have a higher or lower chance of carrying a baby with special needs. Unfortunately for Leona and her partner, Andrew, the test showed that she was in the high-risk group.

'Even at this stage, all I felt was anger and a great resentment towards the doctors, because now we had the worry of whether or not to go ahead with the amniocentesis. We saw a consultant the next day to go over the test results and the possible outcomes of the amnio. Over and over again we asked ourselves whether we could put our baby's life at risk when our journey to get this far had been so long and gruelling.'

Leona and Andrew decided not to go ahead with the amniocentesis, although Cora did, and then found that the time it took for the results to come through were the hardest of her life.

'What if the results were negative but then I had a miscarriage? What would I do if they were positive?'

Two weeks later Cora heard that the results were negative, but the weeks of concern and anxiety marred her memories of her pregnancy.

Richard resented the assumption of the hospital staff that he and his partner Rosemary would not only want the tests, because she was 43, but that they would want a termination if the tests showed that their baby was likely to have a disability:

'We would never have a termination – it goes against all our beliefs. We initially considered having an amnio, but the attitude we met was, "Why bother to have the test if you won't terminate?" We could have tried to explain that it would give us a chance to come to terms with any disability our child might have, but we felt we might be pressured into having a termination if there was a high risk, so in the end we didn't go ahead.'

Caitlin, who had conceived through her third attempt at IVF, specifically told her consultant at the outset of her antenatal care that she didn't want any tests and asked him to make sure that she wasn't subsequently offered them.

'He was very understanding of our feelings and appreciated the reasons for our decision. We wanted this baby, whether the baby was "perfect" or not. To us, our baby would always be perfect.'

There are some rare complications which can arise from some antenatal tests, so if you are offered these, make sure that you are given all the relevant, up-to-date information about the risks and benefits before you decide whether to go ahead with the procedure.

SELECTIVE REDUCTION

This is something you might be offered if you have a multiple pregnancy and there's doubt that you will be able to carry all the babies to term. It may also be offered if antenatal tests show an abnormality in one of the babies. Even when you're convinced it's in everyone's best interests this is probably one of the most stressful and distressing experiences a couple will ever have to undergo, especially as the procedure carries a risk of miscarriage. Some couples who have a selective reduction lose all the babies the woman was carrying anyway, although these risks are smaller than those of continuing with a high-multiple pregnancy. You will want as much information as you can before making your decision, and support throughout.

THE BIRTH

Parents who have had infertility treatment are more prone to accept medical intervention during pregnancy and labour. Perhaps because they have become more used to medical management through the process of assisted conception, it feels natural to continue that medical management now and see the child safely born. Perhaps anxiety levels, on the part of both parent and consultant, are higher, too.

Alison, who had a labour with a high level of intervention, felt that the experience was 'a bit grim' and not what they had planned.

'We'd been through all the NCT antenatal classes and were going to have a natural birth. Instead we ended up with a room full of obstetricians.'

Nevertheless, even if you do have a caesarean or other intervention, most couples agree that in the end it doesn't matter how the baby gets here. Even a caesarean can be a joyous event. Sara had a room full of medical staff for hers, which had been planned because she was suffering from pre-eclampsia.

'Our consultant said, "This is a very precious baby and I want to deliver him for you." And she brought the whole team who had

supported us over all our years of infertility treatment into the operating
theatre, so it was a very jubilant occasion.'

THE LONG-AWAITED BABY

Many, many parents will find every moment with their new baby a
constant and miraculous joy. Donna says:

'I look at Holly and just feel incredibly lucky. Can other parents feel like
this? Here's the baby we thought we would never have, living proof that
miracles do sometimes happen, and I still can hardly believe she's ours.'

Caitlin, too, thinks that

'Even on the bad days, we're so happy.'

If you've spent years trying to have a child, adjusting to the reality
of that child can take some time. As Gilli says:

'By the time a baby is finally here, the idea has built up so much that
the reality can bring you down to earth with a bump. How can
coming to terms with the responsibilities of parenthood ever hope to
live up to those rosy dreams of pastel babygros and broderie anglaise
buggies?'

Rachel feels something similar:

'I spent seven years dreaming – seven years gazing at other people's
lives, wanting a baby of my own. When you've spent seven years in
dreamland, you're much less prepared for reality.'

SPECIAL CARE

It's often harder to get to know and love a baby who needs special
care, simply because there may be physical barriers which prevent

you holding and cuddling your child, and often because you don't yet know whether he or she will make it, which can make it harder for you to decide whether to plan to take the baby home. Jackie, whose twin girls needed special care when they were born early, looks back on the two weeks they spent in the special care baby unit as 'a kind of waiting room'. Although they are now five and both healthy and happy, Jackie still remembers how emotionally draining those two weeks were.

'Everything was on hold. I wanted to spend as much time there with them as I could, but I felt so helpless. There seemed to be very little I could do except wait, pray, wait and see . . .'

If your baby or babies need special care, you may find it helpful to contact one of the support groups that can offer information and advice to parents in this situation. They can help you not only to understand the frightening array of equipment on which your baby's life depends, but also to plan for the day you can take your baby home.

BREASTFEEDING

The benefits of breastfeeding are now so well established that many parents will want to feed their child in this way, yet it doesn't always come easily, as Sara has just discovered.

'When Thomas was born, he was so dozy and little he wouldn't feed from me at all. I was very distressed when he wouldn't.'

Alison, too, tried breastfeeding,

'But he was all doped up and he wasn't having any. It was a let-down, and disappointing, but not something that mattered greatly in the long term.'

Sara was more determined:

'Even now he's seven weeks old, I'm using the breast pump and expressing five or six times a day although I'm still getting very little milk. I want it to work. I keep thinking, this is the one thing I can do naturally.'

If you have had a managed birth, as couples who have been through infertility treatment are more likely to do, it may be more difficult to establish breastfeeding; certainly pethidine can interfere with success. Deborah ran into troubles when her son Matthew was two days old.

'They had to put a tube down him as he'd become severely hypoglycaemic. Luckily for me, one of the midwives at the hospital was also my breastfeeding counsellor, and I felt safe that she was there and reassured me that they had to do this. I felt, from what she said, that this wasn't going to undermine breastfeeding for ever, which I was glad about because it was very important for me to try to make it work.'

There's no theoretical reason why women who have had a caesarean shouldn't be able to breastfeed just as easily as those who have delivered naturally, but circumstances often conspire against it. You will be in hospital longer and find it more difficult to pick up your baby, while staff might be busy and find it hard to help you . . . And unless breastfeeding in those first few days is managed with skill, it's easy for caesarean mothers to get discouraged and give up. The advice of Jane, an experienced NCT breastfeeding counsellor, is to 'ring the bell regardless' if you need the staff to help you establish feeding. Sara is right: this is one thing you can do naturally, and if it's important to you, ask for help.

Parents of multiples are often at a disadvantage, being made to feel that breastfeeding two or more must be an enormous task with little hope of success. As Sophie says,

'They said to me, "Well, there's no harm in seeing how you get on," which made me feel from the start that they didn't expect me to get on very well.'

Uncertainty is often compounded because few of us will ever have seen a mother feeding two babies at one time. Yet many mothers of twins do successfully breastfeed, and even higher multiples may all be partially breastfed.

If you are expecting twins or more and hope to breastfeed your babies, try to spend time with another twin mother before the birth and find out how she manages. It may help you to make some decisions about whether to feed them separately or together, for example, and give you some ideas about practical ways of coping.

PARENTING

Many parents who have had a baby after treatment for infertility find that they have a perspective on birth and parenthood that 'ordinary parents' never have. Sireen says,

'I have no doubts, no doubts at all that we are much better parents because we had to wait so long to have a baby. We're stronger, more positive . . . We appreciate what we have. People who have children without waiting, without any treatment, they just don't know how lucky they are, and we do. I don't think that will ever change.'

Marjorie, who had her first baby at 42 after prolonged treatment for infertility, doesn't find anything to regret in the fact that she was classed as an 'elderly' first-time mother.

'I can honestly say that I'm a much better mother now than I would have been if a baby had popped out with no trouble when I was 22. I've got a perspective on life that I never had then, and I also know how precious this baby is.'

Gilli admits that her feelings are more mixed:

'Not that Callum isn't absolutely wonderful, but at times I feel so guilty if I don't enjoy every second of it. After he was born, I was left with so much grief for the lost years during treatment when I had no energy for anything else. When I was successful and had my baby, I couldn't focus on him fully because of all the grief I was still carrying.'

Taking time to feel you are a family isn't unusual. Perhaps one extra pressure on you, if it's taken you a long time to conceive your first child, is that you may not have much time for reflection if you're considering siblings. Although Thomas is only seven weeks old, Sara knows this is something she and David will have to think about soon.

'I'm content with just Thomas at the moment, but I'm 43 now, and we've got no close family members, and we're very aware that if anything happens to us he'll be on his own, which is a worry for us. I know I couldn't get treatment here now because of the age limit, so I don't know . . .'

Even miracle babies cry

The arrival of a baby is always stressful for any couple, but when you've spent possibly years trying to conceive, when you've invested a great deal of time, money and emotional energy into having a family, how can you possibly admit that some days it all gets a bit much?

During the early months of parenthood, many couples need extra support and, Hope now realises, she and Martin felt more vulnerable about asking for it:

'We were so certain we were going to be perfect parents that we couldn't even admit to one another for ages how difficult we were finding it. Sam had three-month colic, we never got any sleep, he seemed to be so

unhappy to be here . . . It took us a long time to settle down as a family. I think that if we'd been able to admit we were having difficulties, some of the tension might have been taken away. But we couldn't do that.'

Alice says,

'I kept quiet about how I was feeling for weeks and weeks. At my six-week check, I made a special effort to put make-up on and smile. I had this underlying fear that if the doctor saw how bad I felt, he'd take the baby away as I obviously wasn't being a good-enough parent.'

Postnatal depression affects approximately one in ten women who give birth, and those who have given birth via assisted conception aren't immune. In fact, they may find the experience even more terrifying because, after all, they *ought* to be happy now that their dream has come true.

Postnatal depression isn't a sign of being a bad mother, nor of being a parent who can't cope. It's something many mothers experience, partly through the simple turmoil of hormones, although it does seem more difficult for parents to seek help during the demands of early parenthood if they have had a child after treatment for infertility.

Similarly, parents who have had their child through fertility treatment will experience the same stresses on their relationship as a couple as any ordinary parents, and experience the same difficulties. There's always a conflict between being a partner and being a parent, and when you have both focused on being a parent for so long, it's harder to remember how to be a partner, too.

Gilli feels that there are still, stresses and strains in her relationship with her partner,

'But Callum arrived before we had been pushed to our limits. And when I look at this gorgeous little person we've created, I know it's all been worthwhile.'

From baby to toddler to child

Parents who have been the successful beneficiaries of fertility treatment sometimes risk becoming over-protective of their growing children. Grace, whose daughter Abby was born after her sixth IVF attempt, says:

'From the moment Abby was born I could hardly bear to let her out of my sight. I knew that this might be the only child I would ever have and I was determined not only to be with her every moment I could, but to make sure nothing happened to her.'

As Gilli confirms:

'They're so terribly precious when you've tried so hard and you know you might not have any more. It's very frightening, even though it's wonderful.'

Indira, too, whose three-year-old twins were born through IVF, sees other parents running risks she dare not take:

'I see other children walking through the shopping centre where I go and I would never let mine do that. They're always strapped in their buggy or, if I've just got one of the boys with me, he's got his reins on. Even when we go to the park, I'm in a panic the whole time in case one of them falls off the slide and bangs his head, or gets hit by a swing . . . I know I've got to find a balance between keeping them safe and letting them run free, but it's very difficult.'

The increasing success rates of fertility treatments mean that more and more parents are raising babies born through assisted conception techniques. As their experience becomes more widespread, perhaps it will be easier for future parents to find this balance, although it is one that 'ordinary' parents struggle with as well.

THE FUTURE

It's easy to forget how new techniques like IVF are. The first 'test-tube baby', Louise Brown, was born in 1978. The very fact that research into the long-term effects of assisted conception on the children themselves is at an early stage is a source of worry for some parents. Indira says,

'I'll feel happier when Louise Brown herself has healthy children.'

Research into the long-term development of 'high-tech' babies continues, and it will be many years before any conclusions can be drawn. As Sara says,

'Right now I just worry about the effect on Thomas of all the hormones I've taken. Part of me would have been happier if he'd been a girl. But I can't do anything but wait and see. In 20, 30, 40 years' time . . . who's to say what the research will show?'

How much will you tell family and friends about how your child was conceived? How much will you tell your child about its own genesis? The passing of the Human Fertilisation and Embryology Act in the UK in 1990 made it possible for any child born after that date to find out from the HFEA, on reaching the age of 18, whether they were conceived through IVF, or whether their conception involved a donated egg, sperm or embryo. Most parents will have no qualms in sharing every detail with family, friends and the child. After all, this does seem like a miracle. Others may prefer to keep their story to themselves.

Even so, there are oddities you may not be able to avoid, as Sara tells:

'We discovered that David's firm's private health insurance scheme specifically excludes cover for children born through IVF, so we couldn't get private health cover for Thomas there even if we wanted to.'

Janice is nothing but positive when she looks to the future:

'I'm a mother at last, as I always wanted to be. Lily will always know how much she was wanted. I have so much gratitude for everyone who made my dream come true.'

12

When Treatment
Doesn't Result in a Pregnancy

Liz, whose first treatment cycle for IVF has not resulted in a pregnancy, is finding it hard to deal with her emotions:

'It hasn't worked this time, and I was sure it would work. I feel so defeated when I think that I may never feel a child growing inside me. I know I should feel fulfilled in all the other things in my life, but. . . . Why do I need to be a mother? I don't know, but I do. There's something missing.'

Similarly Robin and his partner Erin have just heard that their third, and final, IVF treatment has not worked:

'We are two very work-orientated people. We've always believed that if you worked hard enough at something, you'd eventually achieve it. To be part of a failure is difficult to accept.'

Unfortunately, the link between trying to have children and not having children is not achieved through effort or dedication. As Erin puts it,

'If trying really hard was all it took, I'd have ten children by now.'

Liz, too, feels a sense of having failed:

'Even the photographs of the IVF babies on the walls of the clinic are a reminder that I don't quite measure up.'

Eilish has not yet given up hope.

'I still dream of the day when I will take that test and it will be positive. I see it happening – I can imagine it happening.'

Gilli, looking back, thinks that:

'I wasn't a very nice person to know at that time, but I was suffering so deeply that I couldn't seem to lift myself out of it.'

Depression can be intense, as Liz explains:

'I hope and I dream and I wish . . . Some days I feel I don't want to be here if I'm never going to have a baby.'

If your treatment hasn't resulted in a pregnancy, your clinic should offer you advice and counselling and this can be a useful chance to talk things through. Anger, sadness and frustration are almost inevitable when you and your partner have so much invested, emotionally, personally – and possibly financially – in a successful outcome, and you need an outlet to express your emotions. You may also need time to adjust and recoup your strength before deciding what to do next.

There are several options. You may decide to:

- try again
- try a different type of treatment
- try a different doctor or clinic
- withdraw from further treatment

It might be useful to ask your clinic how many cycles of treatment they usually give before further investigations are undertaken or other forms of treatment are recommended.

Marion says,

'I knew as soon as the test came back negative that we'd try again. I'd come too far down the road to just give up now. I knew we could have two more attempts and I was going to have both of those attempts. If they failed, well, I'd think about that then.'

Callie, after three disappointing IVF cycles, is unable to decide what to do next.

'In a way I'd like to stop. I'm carrying around so many worries and hopes and expectations that I'd like to leave all that behind. But if it means we'll never have children, then I'm not sure I can do that.'

Lena and her partner Tony have been having infertility treatment for four years. They have just heard that their second IVF/ICSI treatment has been unsuccessful, but they have decided to postpone the third, as Lena explains:

'We've decided that we need a break. We need to get things in perspective and get away from this stress for a while. Tony thinks that we're in danger of forgetting that there are other important things in life, and I think he's right. This summer, we're going to have a holiday. It's money we could have spent on the next IVF treatment, but we're putting that money into our relationship, which is just as important. A break to allow us to recharge our batteries makes more sense now than battling straight on.'

Caroline and Paul have decided to take a break for another reason.

'We've been having the most awful rows and taking things out on each other. Our patience has all gone, and emotionally and physically we're at an all-time low. This isn't the right time to go into the next treatment because I think I'd lose my sanity.'

DECIDING TO DISCONTINUE TREATMENT

'I've been struggling with infertility for 12 years now, and know I now need to move on and find a life after endless treatments. But it's so hard to know when to say, "Enough is enough." After all, it means abandoning all my hopes and dreams'.

Ellen has just decided to stop treatment, a decision that Tanya cannot bring herself to make:

'If we stop treatment, it means that I finally have to accept that I will never experience the joys of having children of my own. All of my life I have truly believed that my purpose for being here was to have children. There has never been anything that I've ever wanted more.'

How can you decide when to stop? Many couples speak of the lingering feeling that maybe the next treatment would be the one that finally worked, especially when there are constant new techniques which seem to be able to help couples, even those who have experienced repeated failures. This is something that Kate remembers:

'Making a firm decision to break with DI was a harrowing process. We gradually lost hope of the DI succeeding and the strain of it all took a heavy toll. It felt as though years had been wasted on a dead-end street. We knew couples who had adopted: these were flesh-and-blood children, not a mental image. Were we chasing a mirage? During a holiday, we faced our feelings of failure and emptiness. When we came back home, we crawled back on to the treadmill of treatment and the rollercoaster of emotions, but in the end we were too burnt-out to drag ourselves to hospital any longer. We were thankful for the support of a hospital social worker who helped us to consider the options realistically. Even so, when we put DI behind us it was not in a well-adjusted manner, but with a strong sense of regret and the bitter knowledge that, had we continued, I might have conceived the next month, or the next,

or the one after. . . . But gradually we were able to relax again. The awful obsession with bodily changes which is a feature of all fertility treatments slowly ceased and we began to look to the future.'

If you are considering adoption, as Kate and her partner did, you will need to make a definite decision to stop treatment. Most agencies will refuse to consider you as potential parents if you are still having treatment in case you get pregnant and decide you don't want to pursue the adoption route, and you may find that some even insist you wait for a while afterwards, as Jayne found:

'One agency said that we not only had to give up treatment but that we would then have to grieve for a year. We did apply to foster when we were having treatment, so we were assessed for that, and then when we had given up treatment we went through another two years of assessment to see if we could adopt, although we were initially told it would only take three months as we had been previously assessed for fostering.'

Sara felt that she had more control over whether to continue with treatment or not because she was a private patient.

'I've had both NHS and private treatment and I do think that when you're a private patient they let you make the decisions more. I felt that if ever there was a hope, they would treat us.'

Sara and David were lucky in that they could afford private treatment, and could continue to afford it for the 14 years it took to have their son. Sara says,

'When I look back and add it all up, I reckon that we must have spent over £50,000, not that we begrudge a penny of it. But not everyone can afford to keep going on. Our consultant at one point actually saw our ability to pay for more treatment as a problem. She said, "If you hadn't

been able to afford it, you would have been able to accept the fact that
you can't have a baby long ago." But we didn't accept that, and I'm
glad we didn't.'

Like Sara and David, some couples will want to pursue every
avenue open. Others set their own limits at an early stage of the
treatment, while yet others simply reach a point at which they
cannot afford it any more – either financially or emotionally – and
give up the long struggle. Trish says,

'It seems very harsh to put it in these terms, but we've had four goes at
IVF now and have spent about £12,000, and I just don't think we can
pay for any more. If it was certain, then yes. But it's a treatment where
we've still only got a 50/50 chance that it will work.'

Trish and Michael considered other options beyond IVF, including
surrogacy, but decided that this was not for them. Trish thinks
that,

'You have to find the thing that works for you, and if that's surrogacy,
that's fine, but I knew, once we'd got the information pack and read up
about it, that I couldn't handle what it involved.'

Michael still looks back on his and Trish's decision to stop treatment with mixed feelings:

'I say it was our choice, but "choice" implies that you get something you
want. We didn't get what we wanted. We didn't choose not to have a
child.'

Matt, too, found that not everyone could understand the grief that
he was experiencing:

'So many people – and I think they're just trying to be kind – told me
that children were "over-rated" and that their lives were so much better

before they had children. I think they sometimes envy us, but can't understand how much we envy them.'

Colleen is now 42 and has decided not to have any more treatment for secondary infertility:

'There comes a time when you have to make a decision to give up. The treatment has been so stressful, especially during this past year. I went through extreme mood swings and some very stressful times with my partner, and I wanted to stop this idea of having a second child ruling my whole life. I've sold the pram and given away all the baby things. We had a sailing holiday this year, which was wonderful, and that's not something we would have been able to do if we were still having treatment – or, indeed, if we had a new baby. It doesn't mean I don't have some regrets, but I want to get on with life again.'

Lucy, who has a son and doesn't seem able to conceive again, is also stoical about her situation.

'You deal with what fate hands out to you. What else can you do? I have a lovely little boy. There's an ache inside, but it will pass.'

Moira too has put her 'quest' behind her.

'I don't regret the years we did spend trying to have children. But I don't regret deciding not to follow that road any further. There comes a point where you have to put all of your hope and faith into the rest of your life.'

DECIDING TO ADOPT

The aim of adoption is to provide a family for a child who needs one, with the child's needs and interests coming first. Adoption is not a 'solution' to infertility because the couple will still be infertile, yet adopting a child does offer many couples the chance to nurture and bring up one or more children. For this reason, adoption is a course some couples consider when it becomes clear that they are unlikely to have children any other way.

This is not a book about the relationship between an adopted child and adoptive parents, as that is a lifelong journey which demands – and has been given – entire books devoted to the subject. But it does make sense here to look at the way consideration of adoption fits into a couple's emotional and psychological journey through infertility treatment. Although it may not be the place they thought they were going to reach when they started treatment, many couples do find themselves arriving at a point where adopting a child seems the right thing, as Kate did:

'I cannot say how we would have got through the time after I stopped infertility treatment without the knowledge that an adoption application lay ahead. That in itself proved an emotional minefield, and we had to fight every inch of the way to be accepted, but it's now sixteen years since we left behind the treadmill of infertility treatments, and the emptiness of our childless years is a distant nightmare. We consider ourselves profoundly blessed to have our adopted son and daughter.'

Teresa says,

'When we decided to look into adoption it wasn't because we saw taking someone else's baby as a lesser substitute for having our own baby. It was because we genuinely felt we had "leftover" love to give.'

Janice has many of the same feelings:

'After eight years of infertility we accepted that it just wasn't going to happen for us, and came to terms with the idea that maybe our role in life was going to be as parents in another way. We adopted a brother and a sister, both under five. They were, and still are, beautiful beyond

description, and they are "ours" in every sense of the word that matters.'

Kate echoes this sentiment:

'David was ten weeks old when we adopted him, and from the moment I carried him into our house he was "my baby". He was our own long-awaited child.'

Unofficial adoption has existed for centuries, and it is still the case that some children are brought up by aunts and uncles or grandparents. But most formal adoptions are arranged through agencies, and a couple who wish to adopt a child will find themselves going through a barrage of assessments that can be daunting, stressful and frustrating. There are more parents seeking to adopt than there are babies who need adopting. Agencies have developed rigorous assessment criteria for would-be adoptive parents; many couples are rejected as 'unsuitable', leaving them hurt and confused. Often couples spend years undergoing fertility treatments, so that by the time they come to terms with the fact that they will never have biological children, they are considered too old to adopt.

After seven years of treatment, Jayne and Mark decided to look into adoption.

'We didn't feel the need to have our own genetic child, so tried to adopt, thinking that we would have a good chance of being able to adopt a sibling group. We weren't desperate to have a baby, or even a toddler, because the baby stage is over so quickly anyway. And we thought that if we were given a baby, it might be the only one we ever had. We wanted a family.'

They found the process of 'the adoption lottery' very frustrating.

'It went on and on and on. We had to write essays on our thoughts about our philosophy of child-rearing, children's eating habits, our

relatives. . . . We had over 30 interviews and I felt all the time that they were trying to provoke us into saying the wrong thing. They asked us what we'd do if we were turned down and we said we'd go to another agency, and then we thought maybe we shouldn't have said we'd go to another agency. Every time they went away, we wondered whether we'd said the right thing. Mark said he wouldn't go through it again. I was emotionally drained at the end of it and close to a nervous breakdown.'

Jayne felt they were being judged on their social circumstances.

'During our years of infertility we had built up a nice home, and we were quite shocked to find that this counted against us. They looked at our house, which was neat and tidy, our nice clothes, our holidays – and said it had implications for the sort of child we might be able to adopt. We must be able to take the most difficult children. They said, "These children might leave school without any qualifications. Mightn't you think that one of your own would have gone to university?" No, but how could we persuade them of that?'

Colette almost changed her mind when subjected to the procedures and visits of her local council's social services department:

'I found all the home visits by social workers and everyone quite intrusive and quite demeaning. People who just have children naturally don't have officials come round to their houses first to see if they are suitable. But in my logical moments I knew this had to be the way. If I were a mother placing my baby for adoption, I would want to know that she was going to a good home and to good people.'

Jayne and Mark were initially turned down by their adoption agency.

'They don't even have to give a reason for turning you down, but when we asked, we were told that we wanted a child too much and that we

had not come to terms with our childlessness. They said, "We'll tell you when you're ready and we don't think you're ready yet." And then later, when I said my mum had got terminal cancer – because you have to tell them if there's a change in your circumstances – they said they couldn't approve us while she was still alive because they didn't know how we'd cope with the bereavement, and then we'd have to wait for a year after that to see how we were coping. At that point we put ourselves on the waiting list for a surrogate.'

Although Jayne and Mark were eventually approved for adoption, by then their surrogate mother was pregnant. Their experience shows that, with the best will in the world on both sides, trying to adopt a family can be a difficult and stressful process.

Colette, who did eventually adopt a sibling group, understands why adoption agencies have to be thorough and responsible in their vetting process but adds that the wait can be very frustrating.

'It sometimes seemed to me that they were getting very exercised about small things while there were children sitting having a miserable time in a home somewhere.'

One of the hardest things to come to terms with, if you want to adopt, is knowing that you have so much love to give, and that there are so many children in the world who need a loving family – and yet you can't bring the two together. This is one reason why some couples look into adopting a child from overseas, as Beth and Danny are doing.

'We were told we were too old to adopt here, but we don't believe we're unsuitable parents. The most daunting thing is getting to grips with the paperwork, but we've been through three miscarriages, so many infertility treatments, taken so many different hormones, tried every therapy you can think of. . . . It doesn't matter how many forms they ask us to fill in, it seems easy by comparison.'

The number of parents hoping to adopt from overseas is rising, and you can find help – which you will need – if this is something you want to do. At the back of the book there are details of organisations which can give you information, and you can also find helpful advice online if you have a Internet connection.

Most couples who consider adoption think automatically of a baby coming into the house. For a few lucky couples this will indeed be the case, but if you aren't prepared to consider an older child you may have a very long wait. Changing social patterns mean that unmarried mothers give their babies up for adoption far less frequently than they used to. Yet there are many older children, as well as babies with disabilities, who need a new family.

Pippa doesn't think that, because her son Josh came to her when he was three, their bond is any less strong:

'A tiny baby is a wonder to behold, and I've always felt it was very special seeing and holding my nieces and nephews in those very early days, when they seem so "new", but a child's love is not determined by just that short period of time. An older child can bond with you, and you with the child. It just takes time and a great deal of patience.'

She has sometimes been rebuffed when she mentioned adoption to other infertile couples.

'I didn't mean to hurt them or insult them when I asked if they were considering adoption. Mainly, I wanted to open their eyes to a chance to share the delight that we have gained. And, I think, to help alleviate their pain.'

If you have decided between you that you want to adopt a child, the first thing to do is to contact your local adoption agencies. The British Agencies for Adoption and Fostering (see p. 287) keep lists of addresses and telephone numbers and you can then write giving details about yourself. If you start the process of applying to adopt, there is no guarantee that you will ever be matched with a child who needs a family – but, if everything does work out, you will have the happiness of knowing that a child who needed parents has been placed with parents who needed a child.

Kate feels that

'Adoption is hard work and it never goes away. Your child will always be working through it and so will you.'

For this reason, adoption isn't right for everyone. It presents great challenges along with its joys, and not every couple will feel that it is something they are emotionally equipped to do. If you do adopt, however, you may come to feel as Kate did:

'Of all the things I have done, it is the thing about which I have the least regrets.'

LIVING WITHOUT CHILDREN

'I have a wonderful marriage, a house of the sort I always wanted, enough money to be very comfortable, a loving and supportive family, I enjoy my job, I love my friends. In fact, I have everything a person could ask for, except . . . .'

Ellen is just coming to terms with the fact that she and her husband will never have children. The pain can be intense, as she explains:

'There are so many things that other people take for granted that I long for and will never experience. Feeling a child growing inside me. Hearing my child cry for the first time. Some days, children seem to be all around me and I can't get that hurt out of my mind.'

Coral, too, is resigned to the fact, but on some days finds it difficult to bear.

'*It's awful to walk through a supermarket and hear parents yelling at their child. Or the days I turn on the radio and hear news of parents harming their child. Why should they have children they cannot care for, and I can't?*'

Ellen feels, above everything else, angry:

'*I feel extremely angry and bitter, with myself, with everyone. For years I couldn't get on with my life because my life was on hold while we were waiting for our baby to arrive. And now I'm supposed to sweep all those years under the carpet and start again.*'

It's a feeling Gilli sometimes shares:

'*There's a line from a John Lennon song – "Life is something that happens while you're busy making other plans". How true that is. My life happened without me noticing it. I thought I was in control of everything, but now I realise that I'm not and I wasn't.*'

Coral says,

'*I really envy couples who decided not to have children. It makes me think that they have an all-fulfilling love that leaves no room for other people. I wonder if that means we don't measure up in another way – that Simon and I simply weren't enough for each other. We did look to start a family. Now that children of our own won't just happen for us, we're looking at our relationship all over again and considering the future. I think we'll stay together because we've supported each other through this, but we're looking at a different landscape, and it will take us time to adjust to that.*'

Coming to terms with the fact that you will never have a biological child means working through some strong and painful feelings, and the process may not ever be considered 'closed'. Coral has an honest, if bleak, assessment of the place she has been brought to:

'I don't talk about it any more, and gradually my friends and family will come to believe that this is something I chose. I will know I didn't. If you want to know how I think of myself, then I will always say that I am a childless mother.'

People who wanted children and have to face the fact that they won't have then need time to heal. Sometimes they will need to withdraw into themselves, at others they will need strong support. If you have spent years on the path of fertility treatments, it may take you a while to accept that you need to move to a different path in life and find a different set of values. It may be even harder to accept that those values will one day feel fulfilling – although couples who have been through this transition say it *does* happen, albeit, slowly, and there are positive outcomes after all.

Ray thinks that the experience of infertility has reaffirmed his relationship with his partner, Helia.

'The things we went through only made us stronger – either individually, or as a couple – but we couldn't see that while we were going through it.'

Afterword

'm one of the lucky ones. With my partner, Peter, I have a son and a daughter. A final word, therefore, on how this book came about, as some readers will probably be wondering how someone who has had children would want to write about the pain of not having children, or indeed *could* write about it. So this is my own story.

I always wanted to have a family. From the earliest days I can remember, I dreamed of having a baby of my own. Whether this was instinct or conditioning or fantasy, I didn't care then and I don't care now. All I know is that nothing else mattered.

Instead, I had an ectopic pregnancy which not only took away the child I had longed for but reduced my chances of ever conceiving again. Four years later, I had a miscarriage. Despite everything I could do, my own body seemed to be betraying me. Then . . . nothing.

I kept my temperature charts for a year and embarked upon that obsession with the daily fluctuations we try so hard to interpret. I took vitamins in precise quantities. I eschewed any food that contained additives. I embarked on a fitness regimen that makes me tired to think of it even now. I went for blood tests, which were spectacularly inconclusive. I went to specialist clinics where the date of the appointment always seemed to coincide with the onset of my most vicious period yet, and I endured the comments of doctors that this was probably a good sign that I was ovulating. I went on religious pilgrimages and prayed. Eventually I was prescribed Clomid, another specialist having concluded that I wasn't ovulating at all . . . and shortly afterwards our son, Ben, was conceived.

Throughout the pregnancy, I could hardly believe it was real. And after he was delivered by emergency caesarean I couldn't take in for a long time that he was real, either.

We then lost another baby. So I know how much, even when you already have one of your own, even when people are telling you to be grateful for the blessings you have got, how much that pain hurts.

When my daughter arrived, three years later but a month early, the special care baby unit team were standing by. Again, a life that we thought was assured suddenly seemed in jeopardy as she was hurried out without delay. Christiane came through the experience with only minor scars and I knew, when she was born, that whatever biological or instinctive force which had driven me so hard for so long was now gone. As mysteriously as it had arrived, it went away again. As I held her in my arms, I knew that our family was complete.

So although I have managed to give birth to my children without the high-tech support that many infertile couples need, I know exactly what it's like to want children and feel that you may never have them. I know what it's like to wait and lose hope. I know what it's like to go through tests and be reassured that you have plenty of time and there's nothing to worry about . . . and at the same time feel that reassurance isn't what you want when you need your miracle now.

When I was working as Features Editor on the magazine of the National Childbirth Trust, I proposed in an editorial meeting that we cover the subject of infertility and the new developments in assisted conception. As the NCT was perhaps not the most obvious forum for such a debate (by its very nature, most of our members would have given birth to at least one child), I blithely allowed my home telephone number to be published with the request that anyone who felt they could contribute should ring me. I expected a few calls about secondary infertility, and perhaps some interesting stories about antenatal classes after IVF. By the end of the first week after publication, I had received 102 calls and the answering machine expired. Still the calls continued.

The calls were from women, and some men, whose babies had been born through assisted conception techniques and who wanted to share their experiences of tests, treatments and funding difficulties. They were from couples who had had one child but seemed unable to have another. They were from women currently undergoing treatment who were often isolated and only rarely in good support networks. And they were from health professionals who felt that they had something to offer in this debate.

In talking to the people who called, I was struck my how many of them hadn't felt able to share with friends or family the fact that they were having treatment for their infertility. It was too painful to discuss. No one could really understand how they felt. Sometimes they couldn't explain how it felt. It seemed that the inability to have a child really was, in this day and age, the last secret. Couples didn't tell other people that they were trying to have children, that they were having tests, what those tests felt like, what it was like to live in the land of obsession and hope, what it was like to consider egg donation or surrogacy. . . . And so the idea for the book was born.

You may decide to enlist the support of medical technology to achieve the family you so want to have. You may decide that gamete donation or surrogacy or adoption are the ways forward for you. You may have to fight a battle to get the treatment you want and need. I hope that reading about other people's histories, treatments, successes and failures will make you feel less alone with your feelings as you go through this journey, and may help you to make sense of those strange, swirling emotions that so often seem pushed to one side once we are embarked upon the quest to have children.

More than anything, I hope this book stops you making that strange transition from 'an ordinary couple who seem to be taking longer than usual to conceive' to the 'patients' you may find you become when treatment begins.

You aren't patients, because you aren't 'ill' in the usual sense of the term. What you want is to have a baby, and that's not an illness. If you can stay in charge of the process and feel more informed about what's happening to you, if you can understand what treatments might mean or what various tests will involve, if you can stay a person and not a patient, then no matter where your journey ends, this book will have done what I wanted it to do.

Source Notes

1. Lindblad, A. et al. Effect of nicotine on human fetal blood flow. *Obstetrics and Gynecology*, Vol. 72, No. 3, Part 1, September 1988
2. World Health Organisation criteria
3. HFEA *Sixth Annual Report*, 1997, Table 1, p. 13
4. Hydrosalpinx reduces IVF-Embryo Transfer Implantation Rates. M. R. Freeman, C. M. Whitworth, G. A. Hill. American Society for Reproductive Medicine. http://www.asrm.abstracts
5. Allan Templeton, Joan Morris and Bill Parslow. Factors that affect outcome of in-vitro fertilisation treatment. *Lancet*, November 1996, Vol. 348, Issue 9039, 23
6. Abdallah, H. et al. *British Journal of Obstetrics and Gynaecology*, Obstetric outcome in 232 ovum donation pregnancies. Vol. 105, pp. 332–337, March 1998
7. R. Rai, H. Cohen, M. Dave and L. Regan, Randomised Controlled Trial of Aspirin and Aspirin plus Heparin in Pregnant Women with Recurrent Miscarriage Associated with Phospholipid Antibodies (or Antiphospholipid Antibodies), *British Medical Journal*, 314, 1997, pp. 253–257
8. HFEA *Sixth Annual Report*, 1997
9. HFEA *Sixth Annual Report*, 1997, Table 3, p. 26

Information and Support Organisations

The organisations listed here can provide a wealth of information, advice and support. If you are writing to any of them, please include a stamped addressed envelope as many are charities or very small voluntary groups who rely on fund-raising and donations to continue their work.

This list is not meant to be exhaustive. There are many other charities and organisations which can offer support for a rare disorder or specific syndrome that may be at the heart of your infertility. Your GP is the best starting point for details. Your local library and GP practice noticeboards are also good ways of finding out about support groups and networks which meet in your area.

Every effort has been made to make sure that the information given here is up to date, but addresses, telephone numbers and web site locations inevitably change. If you need more help on a particular topic, first try CHILD or ISSUE as they keep up to date on a wide range of subjects, not only on fertility treatments but on areas such as adoption, egg donation and surrogacy, and keep members informed of new developments.

GENERAL

CHILD
Charter House
43 St Leonard's Road
Bexhill-on-Sea
TN40 1JA
Tel: 01424 732361
Fax: 01424 731858
E-mail: office@email2.child.org.uk
Founded in 1979, this is the national self-help network for those trying for a family. CHILD's members are mainly couples undergoing infertility treatment. The services offered include a telephone helpline open seven days a week, run by volunteers, giving you the chance to talk to someone who has personal experience of infertility. As CHILD's main aim is to support people going through the trauma of infertility, membership is not essential, but members do have access to a range of valuable services, including the quarterly newsletter, *Childchat*, with articles, letters and information, as well as the opportunity to write to a medical adviser for an independent opinion on a particular problem. In addition, CHILD publishes a wide range of factsheets and offers a network of support through local groups.

Human Fertilisation and Embryology Authority (HFEA)
Paxton House
30 Artillery Lane
London E1 7LS
Tel: 0171 377 5077
Fax: 0171 377 1871
The HFEA is the statutory body which regulates assisted reproduction technology and human embryo research. It licenses and monitors all clinics in the UK which carry out IVF, DI and embryo research, and also regulates the storage of gametes and embryos. All licensed clinics must follow the professional, legal and ethical standards set out in the HFEA *Code of Practice*. The HFEA also collects information about licensed treatments and outcomes.

ISSUE – The National Fertility Association
114 Lichfield Street
Walsall,
WS1 1SZ
Tel: 01922 722888
Fax: 01922 740070
E-mail: webmaster@issue.co.uk

Founded in 1976, ISSUE is an information and support service dealing with all aspects of infertility and assisted conception. Working independently of any treatment centre, it can provide a wide range of services to people who experience infertility and those who work with them. Couples who join receive a set of factsheets tailored to their individual circumstances, have access to telephone counselling on medical or emotional problems by professionally trained staff, and can be put in touch with local support groups or other members who are willing to share their experiences on particular aspects of infertility. ISSUE also produces a guide to all UK clinics who offer assisted conception treatments.

PRECONCEPTUAL CARE

Foresight – Association for the Promotion of Preconceptual Care
28 The Paddock
Godalming
GU7 1XD
Tel: 01483 427839
Call for details of how to obtain an information booklet.

HEALTH MATTERS

Daisy Chain – Early Ovarian Failure Support Group
PO Box 230
Barnet
EN5 2BF
Can give support and information to women who have suffered a premature menopause.

The National Endometriosis Society
50 Westminster Palace Gardens
Artillery Row
London SW1P 1RL
Helpline (7pm–10pm daily): 0171 222 2776
Tel: 0171 222 2781
Fax: 0171 222 2786
The national helpline is staffed by trained volunteers, all of whom have endometriosis and so understand its effects from personal experience. It is also for partners and family who may need reassurance and information too. Through local groups and a quarterly newsletter, the society also provides support and information for women diagnosed with endome-

triosis, and you can receive individual replies to medical questions. There is also a wide range of publications, including factsheets on the various types of treatment and a leaflet called *Endometriosis, Fertility, Pregnancy*.

SEEKING TREATMENT

National Infertility Awareness Campaign (NIAC)
PO Box 2106
London W1A 3DZ
Freephone for information pack: 0800 716345
Tel: 0171 439 3067
Fax: 01721 437 0553
NIAC campaigns for fertility services to be made available across the UK in an equitable way so that everyone who needs it has access to treatment. For an information pack on how you can help to campaign for funding and treatment within your health authority, call the free telephone number. NIAC can also give you up-to-date details on which treatments, if any, are available on the NHS in your area, together with information on eligibility criteria, waiting times and the names of hospitals or clinics from which your health authority purchases treatments.

COMPLEMENTARY THERAPIES

Each therapy has its own organisation and register which can help you find a registered and appropriately qualified practitioner in your area. Many complementary therapists can be found in the Yellow Pages (often under 'Clinics'), but try asking around first for a personal recommendation. For more information about complementary therapies, write to the following address.
The British Register of Complementary Practitioners
PO Box 194
London SE16 1QZ

Acupuncture

The British Acupuncture Council
Park House
206–208 Latimer Road
London W10 6RE
Tel: 0181-964 0222

Aromatherapy

International Federation of Aromatherapists
2–4 Chiswick High Road
London W14 1TH
Tel: 0181-742 2605

Herbs

National Institute of Medical Herbalists
56 Longbrook Street
Exeter
EX4 6AH
Tel: 01392 426022

Homeopathy

The British Homeopathic Association
27a Devonshire Street
London W1N 1RJ
Tel: 0171-935 2163

The Society of Homeopaths
2 Artizan Road
Northampton
NN1 4HU
Tel: 01604 621400

Osteopathy

Osteopathic Information Service
PO Box 2074
Reading
RG1 4YR
Tel: 0118 512051

Reflexology

Holistic Association of Reflexologists
92 Sheering Road
Old Harrow
CM17 0JW
Tel: 01279 429060

COUNSELLING

British Association for Counselling
1 Regent Place
Rugby
CV21 2PJ
Tel: 01788 578328
The Association can provide you with details of qualified counsellors working in your area if you send an SAE.

British Infertility Counselling Association
69 Division Street
Sheffield
S1 4GE
BICA provides a nationwide referral system for those who want to talk to a specialist infertility counsellor. Send SAE for details of professional counsellors working in your area.

DONATION

National Gamete Donation Society
Regional IVF Unit
St Mary's Hospital
Whitworth Park
Manchester
M13 0JH
Tel: 0161 276 6000
Fax: 0161 224 0957
The Society aims to raise public awareness of the need for egg and embryo donation, provide potential gamete donors with information about what is involved and tell people which is their nearest treatment centre.

DI Network
PO Box 265
Sheffield
S3 7YX
This is a network of parents of children conceived by donor insemination and those contemplating or undergoing treatment. DI Network provides support to existing parents of children conceived by DI, to the children themselves, and to those contemplating DI. A further aim is to increase public awareness and acceptance of DI.

MISCARRIAGE

Clinic Co-ordinator
Recurrent Miscarriage Clinic
St Mary's Hospital
Marylebone Road
London NW1 5YE
You will need to be referred to this clinic by your GP. The clinic mainly offers help to women who have had three or more miscarriages with the same partner.

Miscarriage Association
c/o Clayton Hospital
Northgate
Wakefield
WF1 3JS
Tel: 01924 200799
The Miscarriage Association is a national charity offering support and information on all aspects of pregnancy loss. There is a network of local telephone contacts and support groups throughout the UK, and the Association also publishes leaflets, factsheets and a quarterly newsletter for members. The helpline gives advice and support to women who have had or who are experiencing pregnancy loss.

SANDS (Stillbirth and Neonatal Death Society)
28 Portland Place
London W1N 4DE
Helpline: 0171 436 5881
SANDS offers support to anyone whose child has died during pregnancy or as a young baby. There are local support groups who meet regularly in many areas.

SATFA (Support around Termination for Abnormality)
73–75 Charlotte Street
London W1P 1LB
Helpline: 0171 631 0285
Tel: 0171 631 0280
SATFA is a registered charity which supports parents who have terminated a pregnancy after a diagnosis of abnormality in their baby, or parents who are making the decision whether or not to have a termination. As well as offering a helpline, and providing information on antenatal screening and testing, SATFA provides many local contacts and support groups; call the office number (not the helpline) for details of these.

SURROGACY

COTS (Childlessness Overcome Through Surrogacy)
Loandhu Cottage
Gruids
Lairg
IV27 4EF
Tel: 01549 402777
Information line: 01549 402401
E-mail: cotsuk@enterprise.net
COTS, launched in 1988, is a voluntary organisation assisting both childless couples and surrogates. It is run by people who have all had first-hand experience of surrogacy. COTS is not a commercial surrogacy agency but, with over 750 members and having been involved in over 200 surrogate births, aims to pass on this collective experience for the benefit of others by giving both practical advice and moral support. COTS can help both surrogates and would-be parents to understand the implications of surrogacy before they enter into an arrangement, and will explain how to deal with any problems that may arise. Factsheets and information booklets are available, but please call to check details of current prices. The information line gives an 8-minute recorded message with details of COTS and surrogacy.

Triangle is an offshoot of COTS which introduces intended parents to potential surrogate mothers. Every member of COTS who is actively seeking a surrogate and is within the criteria set by the executive committee automatically becomes a member of Triangle after being seen by a counsellor/mediator. Triangle cannot give any guarantee of ever being able to find a potential surrogate for a couple. It cannot advertise for surrogates, but has to wait for them to contact COTS. While COTS is willing to give general help and advice regarding surrogacy to non-UK couples, limited resources mean that only couples and surrogates living in the UK for the duration of the arrangement can be placed on Triangle's 'active' list.

PARENTING AFTER INFERTILITY

Association for Postnatal Illness
25 Jerdan Place
London SW6 1BE
Tel: 0171-386 0868
The Association for Postnatal Illness offers information and support through one-to-one telephone counselling for anyone undergoing post-natal depression. Telephone for details of a contact in your area. Send an SAE for information and useful leaflets about postnatal illness.

Blisslink/Nippers (Baby Life Support Systems/National Information for Parents of Prematures: Education, Resources, Support)
17–21 Emerald Street
London WC1N 3QL
Tel: (office): 0171-831 9393
Bliss Parent Support Freecall: 0500 618140 weekdays 10.30am – 4.30pm
Blisslink offers support and a listening ear for parents whose babies need intensive or special care. Blisslink can provide factsheets, leaflets, details of local support groups and put you in touch with individual befrienders.

MAMA (Meet-a-Mum Association)
26 Avenue Road
London SE25 4DX
Helpline: 0181-768 0123 weekdays 7pm–10pm
MAMA is a national group which puts mothers in contact with other mothers in their area. They also offer leaflets and a newsletter. The helpline provides a listening ear to mothers with postnatal illness or depression or those who feel lonely and isolated.

NCT (National Childbirth Trust)
Alexandra House
Oldham Terrace
London W3 6NH
Tel: 0181-992 8637
As well as offering social opportunities to meet other new parents in your local area, the NCT runs postnatal exercise classes and discussion groups at which you can talk over your concerns. Look in the phone book under NCT for the name of your local contact, who will be able to give you more

information, or call the number above for details of your local branch. They will also be able to put you in touch with a trained breastfeeding counsellor who lives nearby. All counsellors are mothers who have breastfed their own children. If you are having difficulties with breast-feeding or lack confidence, you may find talking to a breastfeeding counsellor helpful. There is no charge for their support. In addition, many branches run support groups for women who have, or have had, postnatal depression. Some will also be able to put you in touch with other local parents who have had postnatal depression and who can talk to you on a mother-to-mother basis.

TWINS AND MORE

Multiple Births Foundation
Institute of Obstetrics and Gynaecology
Queen Charlotte's Hospital
Goldhawk Road
London W6 0XG
Tel: 0181 383 3519
The Multiple Births Foundation runs regular evening telephone 'clinics' for parents of twins or more, and can offer information and support to expectant parents and those considering infertility treatment.

TAMBA (Twins and Multiple Births Association)
PO Box 30
Little Sutton
L66 1TH
Tel: 0151 348 0020
TAMBA Twinline (for hours see below): 01732 868000
TAMBA has set up a support group for parents expecting twins or more babies following infertility treatment. The group also provides continuing support after the babies are born. TAMBA's other support networks include groups for one-parent families and a special needs group. The Association also produces informative leaflets on feeding multiple babies by both breast and bottle.
  The TAMBA Twinline is a listening and information service open Monday to Friday 7pm–11pm and Saturday and Sunday 10am–11pm. The call will be answered by a parent of twins or more, who can give you up-to-date information on a wide range of issues and support in stressful situations.

FOSTERING AND ADOPTION

National Foster Care Association
Leonard House
5–7 Marshalsea Road
London SE1 1EP
Tel: 0171 828 6266

British Agencies for Adoption and Fostering
Skyline House
200 Union Street
London SE1 0LX
Tel: 0171 593 2000
Fax: 0171 593 2001

The Inter-Country Adoption Line
Helpline: 0171 972 4014
Funded by the Department of Health, this helpline offers information about adopting from overseas. It can provide you with advice about the country you hope to adopt from and the legal requirements of which you will need to be aware.

National Organisation for the Counselling of Adoptees and Parents
112 Church Road
Wheatley
OX33 1LU

OASIS
Dan-Y-Graig
Balaclava Road
Glais
Swansea
SA7 9HJ
Tel: 01792 844329
OASIS can give information on adoption from abroad.

Parent to Parent Information on Adoption Services
Lower Boddington
Daventry
NN11 6YB
Tel: 01327 260295
A registered charity which provides advice and encouragement for parents who have adopted children and for long-term foster carers.

Internet Resources

This is not a manual which can tell you everything you need to know about how to get online, or how to cope with every technical problem you may meet (and there are always some) on your way to full access to newsgroups and the worldwide web. However, if you can equip yourself with a computer and a modem, and sign yourself up with an Internet Service Provider (especially one with a truly helpful Help Desk), you will find that the online world can offer you a great deal in the way of support and information. It won't always be easy to find what you are looking for: the net is large, inefficient and variable in quality, and it can take you time to find your way around, even using one of the many search engines. (It's been described as like trying to find what you're looking for in a large library where someone's tipped the books and the catalogue cards all over the floor – and then turned out all the lights.) However, if you are at any stage of infertility treatment – from deciding whether you have a problem, to parenting after IVF, to looking at a child-free future – you will be able to find a great deal of benefit once you've dipped your toes in the water, as each site has links to other web sites and you will eventually end up where you want to be. There is also no doubt that a well-maintained web site can give you more up-to-date information about a topic you're interested in than anything else you can reach in the middle of the night.

WEB SITES

More and more treatment centres in the UK are now publishing details on the web, and although their main intention is commercial they do provide 'add-ons' by way of articles and information. Their pages often include valuable links to other sites of interest where you can follow up a particular topic.

Many American clinics and treatment centres have large web sites. They often publish a wide variety of information which you will find useful, although you must remember that techniques used in the USA and the drug regimes they mention, will vary from those used elsewhere. Also, the business-like attitude to surrogacy and gamete donation reflected in many of these sites mirrors the fact that in the USA surrogacy and egg and sperm donations can be purely commercial transactions. Very different considerations apply in the UK, as they also do to adoption.

If you're looking for particular information, always check the date the page was last updated (some information goes out of date very quickly), and whether the site is sponsored by a drug company. Always bear in mind that although the Internet is an excellent source of information, in order to be of real use the materials should come from a reputable, impartial source, not from a company with products to sell or someone with an opinion to promote.

Here's a selection of the most accessible and informative sites below; you will find many more once you start looking for yourself.

SUPPORT AND INFORMATION

British Fertility Society
http://www.repromed.org.uk
Information about the latest research plus the contents listing of the most recent issue of the Society's journal.

CHILD
http://www.child.org.uk
Useful information for infertile couples in the UK.

European Infertility Network
http://www.ein.org
A non-profitmaking organisation, disseminating up-to-date information and news about infertility and the work of infertility support associations with a focus on Europe, including the UK, with information about clinics,

treatments and support services. You can also sign up for their free e-mail
updating service.

European Society of Human Reproduction and Embryology
http://ferti.net
This site gives you access to current information and research, enabling
you to find out more about recent research studies and practical developments.

Fertile Thoughts
http://www.fertilethoughts.net
This site contains a variety of sections, including information on infertility,
adoption and surrogacy, as well as pregnancy and bringing up children. 'Just
Starting' is a resource for couples who have just started trying to conceive and
are looking for basic information and support. You can also post queries on
the 'corkboard message centers' for answering by online experts and professionals. The site also includes 'Infertility FAQ for Women of Size', 'Home
Pregnancy Test HCG Levels and Mini-FAQ', 'Ovulation Predictor Kit FAQ',
'Hormone Levels', 'IUI FAQ' and a BBT chart spreadsheet with accompany-
ing Microsoft Excel file for you to print out your own chart templates!

Human Fertilisation and Embryology Authority
http://www.hfea.gov.uk
As well as containing a wide variety of up-to-date information about
treatment and services, this site contains many links that you can follow
up to find out more about topics of particular interest. It also allows you to
download the document 'Choosing a Clinic: Questions and Answers',
which contains a full list of questions that couples should consider asking
if they are contemplating IVF or treatment involving donor eggs or sperm.

INCIID: International Council on Infertility: Information Dissemination
http://www.inciid.org
A large web site from a US non-profit organisation which aims to provide
both information and support. INCIID (pronounced 'Inside') contains
pages of facts and figures on the diagnosis, treatment and prevention of
infertility and pregnancy loss. It's also a good jumping-off point to find out
more about the newsgroups, mailing lists and web sites that might be
most useful and relevant to you.

ISSUE
http://www.issue.co.uk
The ISSUE (National Fertility Association) web site contains information

about current treatments available in the UK and can keep you up to date with new developments. It also lets you know about local groups and the ways in which ISSUE can offer you support.

National Infertility Awareness Campaign
http://www.ivf.net/niac
Information about the work of the campaign plus factsheets from their campaigning pack.

ONNA
http://www.directiondesigns.com/onna
ONNA – as in Oh No! Not (my period) Again! – is an online support group whose web site provides helpful information about conception and self-help for infertility, as well as details of how to subscribe to the ONNA mailing list, and the BabyTwo and OYIP (Oh, Yippee, I'm Pregnant) mailing lists.

Resolve
http://www.resolve.org
The American equivalent of CHILD or ISSUE, this organisation has chapters in most US states. Of interest to those outside the USA are some of the articles it includes on its website, such as 'Infertility Myths and Facts', 'Managing Family and Friends' and 'Coping with the Holidays', a mixture of practical advice and emotional support. It's also a useful place to read discussions on current developments and issues.

TREATMENT CENTRES

Atlanta Reproductive Health Center
http://www.ivf.com
A full and comprehensive site (with a search tool to help you find your way around) put together by Mark Perloe MD. It covers most aspects of infertility, including recurrent miscarriage, a good discussion of the causes and cures of endometriosis, and information about immune-factor treatments. There is an online copy of his book *Miracle Babies and Other Happy Endings*, as well as video clips (for those with high-speed links). The site also includes a very informative paper, 'Male Fertility Overview', a long document (approximately 92K) to download but one that gives a detailed discussion of the assessment and treatment of male factor infertility.

Assisted Conception Unit, University College Hospital, London
http://www.acu-uch.demon.co.uk

A very informative site, including a series of slides taken at the ACU showing the process of ICSI and a four-cell embryo resulting from the procedure.

Assisted Conception Unit, Leeds General Infirmary
http://www.leeds.ac.uk/medicine/res_school/crgd/rmu/welcome.htm
A variety of information, including information about conception (with photographs of a human egg at various stages) and preconceptual care.

The Bridge Centre
http://www.thebridgecentre.co.uk
The home page of this London clinic has an extremely useful and easy-to-follow table outlining the various causes of infertility, with a summary of the investigations that are carried out and the treatment options for each one.

Centre for Reproductive Medicine, University of Bristol
http://www.repromed.org.uk/ndog
The 'Bristol Infertility Pages' provide useful advice on pre-pregnancy care, information regarding infertility and the treatments on offer, including a discussion on choosing between IVF and GIFT, and an Infertility Patient's Directory, plus many links to relevant websites.

Oxford Fertility Unit, Nuffield Department of Obstetrics and Gynaecology
http://www.ox.ac.uk
Much information about IVF, including pictures and videos of ICSI, many other images, and links to other sites.

If you want to know whether a treatment centre you are considering has a website, type their name into one of the many Internet search engines. You may find that they are already online.

ADOPTION

Adoption.com Inc.
http://www.adoption.com
The home pages of this company, 'home to the world's largest online, searchable registry of hopeful adoptive parents', are probably only of practical use to couples in the USA, but if you're interested in adopting overseas you can find some useful information here. There are also personal stories and professional articles, along with a newsletter, although if you're feeling vulnerable, the 'Today's Waiting Child' message may tug too hard at your heartstrings.

MULTIPLES

The Triplet Connection
http://www.tripletconnection.org
An informative and supportive web site for families who have, or are expecting, triplets, quadruplets, quintuplets or more. The Triplet Connection, a non-profit US organisation, has a large database of medical information regarding larger multiple pregnancies and their outcome, including information on selective reduction for those who are faced with this difficult decision, as well as other multiple-birth pregnancy and labour concerns. The pages also include many networking opportunities with other families, some in the UK, who are willing to share their experiences of life with multiple infants to help others know what to expect and what to plan and prepare for, and samples from their quarterly newsletter to read online. The overall message from this site is one of encouragement – that life with multiples can bring challenges, but is also very rewarding.

SURROGACY

COTS
http://www.surrogacy.org.uk
The COTS web site provides information about the process of surrogacy in the UK, its legalities, and information for all those interested in being a surrogate or a parent via surrogacy.

The American Surrogacy Center (TASC)
http://www.surrogacy.com
TASC provides a wealth of information about surrogacy, both traditional (using artificial insemination) and gestational surrogacy, as well as about egg donations, for both donors and recipients. While the site obviously has an extremely American slant, some of the emotional resonances are the same everywhere. There are articles along the lines of 'Is surrogacy right for you?' and others outlining the ways people have dealt with the financial side of surrogacy arrangements. TASC also has a Surrogacy and Egg Donation Message Board where you can post messages or read postings from other people all over the world who have been involved in surrogacy or egg donation.
    A very valuable aspect of the site is the inclusion of the male point of view. Men are encouraged to share their feelings and ask questions relating to any aspect of the process, whether a surrogate is carrying

your baby or you are the husband of a woman who is carrying someone else's baby.

Center for Surrogate Parenting and Egg Donation Inc, Beverly Hills
http://www.surroparenting.com
Although this is an American site, the articles about the experiences of many couples who have created a family through surrogacy, and the experiences of surrogates themselves, make interesting reading.

Surrogate Mothers Online
http://www.SurromomsOnline.com
A web site created by surrogate mothers which aims to be a resource for information, support and friendship to surrogate mothers and potential surrogate mothers as well as to parents and prospective parents via surrogacy. From their home page, you can sign up for their e-mail support groups.

OTHER TOPICS

Endometriosis

http://www.ivf.com/endohtml.html
Extensive information from the Atlanta Reproductive Health Center.

Impotence

http://www.impotence.org/ks/index.html
Although impotence is one of the less common causes of infertility problems, this site, from the American Foundation for Urologic Disease, contains some useful information.

Klinefelter's

http://www.genetic.org/ks/index.html
This web site is maintained by Klinefelter Syndrome and Associates, a US non-profit organisation.

Low-tech ways to help you conceive

http://www.fertilethoughts.net
The site contains the FAQ compiled by Roger A. Hunt, PhD, using

information from several newsgroups, which lists many methods that couples have used to maximise their chances of pregnancy before seeking medical help. (Always check with your GP before making radical changes to your diet, lifestyle or medication.)

Polycystic Ovary Syndrome

http://www.pcosupport.org
PCO Support provides information on the condition, including medical journal articles and links to other sources of support.

Turner's syndrome

http://www.onr.com/ts-texas
Information, links to newsgroups and further resources.

MORE INFORMATION

Fertilitext
http://www.fertilitext.org
While sponsored by drug companies (currently Serono Laboratories, Ferring Pharmaceuticals and Organon, Inc.) and part of the Stadtlanders Pharmacy Website, the stated aim of Fertilitext is to 'provide information about fertility and reproductive issues to those pursuing fertility treatment.' So, if you can ignore the invitations to have the latest drugs delivered direct to your door, you can find out about the latest developments, related web pages, relevant books and articles, an avenue for help on clinical questions, and, naturally, a great deal of up-to-date information about the drugs often used in infertility treatment, which can be very enlightening if you want to know more about something you're taking or have been started on something relatively new.

IHR Infertility Resources
http://www.ihr.com
Information on treatments and drugs, articles about egg donation, and links to other resources.

The *Lancet*
http://www.thelancet.com

The site of this British medical journal can offer you access to research articles about new developments in infertility treatment.

Lifeseek
http://website.lineone.net/~lifeseek
A company that mainly aims to help couples from outside the UK who wish to come here for infertility treatment; the site provides information about clinics, treatment and accommodation.

Pregnancy and Women's Health Information
http://www.womens-health.co.uk
Edited and maintained by Danny Tucker with a view to providing information about all aspects of pregnancy and birth, so that women can make more informed choices about their care and treatment. Topics include: polycystic ovary syndrome, recurrent miscarriage, ectopic pregnancy, screening for Down's syndrome, clomiphene and getting pregnant, and antiphospholipid antibody syndrome and pregnancy.

NEWSGROUPS

If, like me, you find newsgroups hard to access initially, contact your service provider and ask them for help. That is what they are there for. A good question to start with is, 'How can I find out which newsgroups you can give me access to?' because not all the servers carry all the newsgroups – not surprisingly, as there are over twenty-five thousand of them. You may need to configure some settings in your newsreader program before you're up and running. However, don't despair – it can be done (even I did it)! Once you have access to instant, immediate online support, you'll wonder how you ever lived without it.

With so many newsgroups operating, it's not always easy to find the one you're looking for. A good way to find newsgroups which discuss the topic you're interested in is to use one of the search tools (such as DejaNews http://www.dejanews.com or Alta Vista http://www.altavista.digital.com selecting 'search Usenet'). Search for a keyword (such as infertility, endometriosis, miscarriage, and so on). You will then get access to a list of newsgroups which discuss this topic, allowing you instant access to the most recently posted messages. If they're on track for you, you can choose to subscribe to the group. (You can just as easily, of course, unsubscribe later.)

The newsgroup news.announce.newusers contains a lot of useful introductory information about Usenet and newsgroups, as does news.newusers.questions. This may take a while to read, but it will help new users to find their way around much more easily.

Newsgroups do develop their own shorthand, which can take some days to translate. A comprehensive list of acronyms and abbreviations used in newsgroups, which you may find helpful when you first start navigating your way around the oceans of information available, is posted at http://www.fertilethoughts.net and circulates the newsgroups from time to time as baffled newcomers post queries. This can be very helpful for new users – otherwise it may take you a little time to work out that the frequently seen DH stands for 'Darling Husband' or that AF translates as 'Aunt Flo' (AF arrived = my period started).

Because most of the infertility newsgroups are dominated by American contributions, there will be much discussed there that is not relevant to anyone outside the US healthcare system. Questions about insurance issues related to paying for treatments, and personal recommendations of doctors and clinics, may not be pertinent to you, but you can choose not to read those messages when you see them posted. Another thing to remember is that not everyone will have similar views; some people will post deliberately provocative messages and wait for an all-out argument to ensue.

A word of warning if you're thinking of participating in online discussion forums. Commercial companies often monitor Internet traffic and 'harvest' e-mail addresses from messages posted to newsgroups. The companies then use these addresses to send junk e-mails (spam) to you, which can become an unwelcome problem. One way round this is to sign up for one of the news services (such as Deja News, although you will see endless opportunities to avail yourself of free web-mail once you're online); you will be given a free web-based e-mail account and new e-mail address, which you can then use to participate in newsgroups while protecting your permanent e-mail account. This also allows you, if you wish, to protect your own identity as you can participate in newsgroups under a pseudonym. Always think twice before posting personal information about yourself or others. These are open boards: you never know who is reading.

You will also see a lot of messages offering left-over drugs from treatment cycles. Many web sites automatically refuse to post such ads, but some get through in newsgroups. These sales are risky: you have no guarantees as to whether the drugs are genuine or current. Steer clear, however tempting.

As many of the people who are participating in the newsgroups may be at a very vulnerable time in their lives, it's considered polite to include some sort of 'warning' code in the subject line if there's something in the message that may upset someone. For example, (pg) lets people know that the message mentions a pregnancy. This allows others who have supported the person through their infertility treatment to offer their messages of goodwill, but it also allows those whose treatment has just failed, perhaps, to choose not to read that message if they cannot cope with it. You will often see the word (vent) in the subject line – this simply means that someone is 'venting' their feelings, and perhaps expressing some very difficult and negative emotions.

If this prospect sounds daunting, don't let it be. The members of newsgroups were all new once, and the participants change as new members join every day and others leave. Some passing through the alt.infertility newsgroups will graduate to misc.kids.pregnancy, for example. At their best, newsgroups allow you to discuss sensitive issues with a degree of anonymity at any hour of the day.

The following are some of the groups currently active. Not all will suit you in their tone, content or specific interest. However, you can get a flavour of the range and flavour of discussions by 'lurking' for a while – reading the messages that other people post without anyone being aware of your presence. That in itself is enough for some people. Others may want to join in.

alt.infertility
This is a busy and informative newsgroup with a mixture of questions, personal stories and advice pertaining to all issues related to infertility. Subjects range from ways of improving the odds of pregnancy using BBT charts and alternative therapies to being involved in high-tech treatments such as IVF and new areas such as assisted hatching and immunological treatment. It's strong on the emotional stresses and strains, the impact that treatment has on self-image and self-confidence, and on a couple's relationship and wider relationships with family and friends, as well as exploring pregnancy loss after infertility treatment and opting out of treatment to pursue a child-free future.

alt.infertility.alternatives
A newsgroup to help people explore adoption, foster parenting and child-free living as well as moving on from infertility treatment.

alt.infertility.pregnancy
This group provides emotional support for those who have achieved pregnancy after enduring the struggles of infertility. The busiest pregnancy group (misc.kids.pregnancy) cannot always provide an adequate forum for those women, finally pregnant after infertility, who may want to discuss their worries, ambivalent feelings and fears for the future along with all the changes that usually happen in pregnancy.

alt.infertility.primary
The FAQ for this newsgroup establishes this as a place for 'anyone without any living biological children after suffering infertility'. It offers a place where people who do not, and may never have, children can express their unique and often strong feelings about their situation.

alt.infertility.secondary
The main focus of this group is the emotional issues related to secondary infertility, giving people a chance to discuss infertility issues as well as their child or children. While some participants had no previous problems conceiving a child, some had often extensive infertility treatment to achieve their first pregnancy – so parenting after infertility is also a frequent topic.

alt.infertility.surrogacy
Encourages the discussion of all aspects and situations arising from gestational and host surrogacy.

alt.support.diabetes
For everyone diagnosed with or affected by diabetes.

alt.support.endometriosis
Endometriosis is often associated with infertility, and difficulties conceiving are a frequent topic in this newsgroup, along with other concerns for women with endometriosis.

alt.support.pco
PCO (or PCOS) stands for Polycystic Ovary Syndrome. This newsgroup provides information and emotional support for women affected by this endocrinal disorder.

alt.support.turner-syndrome
For all those with or affected by this genetic condition, with contributions from women and girls of all ages, often including information both from Turner's women who are trying to conceive, and those who have managed to get pregnant and raise a family.

misc.health.infertility
This group discusses medical issues related to treating infertility. You may see the same messages appearing here as in alt.infertility (cross-posted), since not all service providers carry the 'alt' (alternative) groups.

sci.med.obgyn
A moderated group, mainly for professionals and researchers, which discusses the science and practice of obstetrics and gynaecology. However, it does allow members of the public to ask general questions related to medical practice in this area.

soc.support.pregnancy.loss
The Charter for this newsgroup states that it aims to provide support and information, in a supportive and non-judgemental way, for anyone experiencing or concerned about the trauma of miscarriage (including blighted ovum), ectopic pregnancy, therapeutic terminations, stillbirth or neonatal death. The web site http://web.co.nz/~katef/sspl includes the soc.support.pregnancy.loss charter.

MAILING LISTS

There are hundreds and thousand of e-mail support groups out there, and some of them have been set up to discuss and help people to deal with particular aspects of infertility. One comprehensive database of current mailing lists is at http://www.liszt.com. It is always a good idea to get more information about a list before you attempt to subscribe, and a database like Liszt will guide you through doing so. The list owners may request further information from you before signing you on, especially if the list deals with a particularly sensitive topic. Once you're signed on, you'll get all the messages from that group (or a digest of them) via your e-mail address.

Many web sites invite you to join their mailing list, but these are usually 'closed' lists (only allowing them to talk to you, and not vice versa). Mailing lists differ from newsgroups in that messages go back and forth via e-mail. Once you're on a list, all the messages sent to the list's central address will appear in your mailbox, and everyone else on the list will receive whatever you send. Most lists are unmoderated, which means that messages received are rebroadcast automatically without any screening. If a list is moderated, it means that a human being somewhere is pruning out irrelevant or inappropriate messages before they are re-sent.

Each list has two addresses:

- *administrative address:* this is the address you need to send your requests to subscribe, unsubscribe, for help and for information
- *list address:* this is where you send your contribution to the discussion

Most lists are now automated (the two main list managers are LISTSERV and MajorDomo) and, once you send your request to subscribe, the automated program will take the return address from your e-mail and add it to the list. You will soon receive a message confirming your subscription, telling you how to post messages and how to unsubscribe from the list; and then you will start to receive e-mail messages from everyone else who has written to the central address. You can choose to reply by posting to the list address so everyone can see your answer, although sometimes you will want to respond just to individuals – perhaps if they have sent a specific question to which you know the answer, or because they've asked for support and you just want to let them know you've been there too.

Many lists allow you to subscribe anonymously – no one except the list owner will know you're there. This allows you to browse through the messages and get a feel for the group before committing yourself to joining in. Lurking is perfectly acceptable. But once you do post a message, obviously you can't keep your presence a secret any longer.

The list owners will send you an e-mail which tells you how to unsubscribe – don't lose it. Many lists are very heavy in traffic, and if you go away for a few days your mailbox may contain several hundred messages by the time you get back. You can unsubscribe – leave the list for a while when you're away – and resubscribe when you return.

The following are some of the mailing lists currently operating. Not all the addresses will still work as lists, however, and their servers change constantly. However, it will give you an idea of the range and specificity of what is on offer and start you off on a search for a list that will offer you the support you are looking for.

BabyTwo
For those who want to discuss the specific effects of secondary infertility. For more information visit the BabyTwo home page at: http/:www.geocities.com/Heartland/Prairie/2874/index.html

DI Support
A group, monitored by Valerie Singer, for people undergoing or considering donor insemination or donor in-vitro fertilisation. To subscribe, send a message to external-majordomo@palladium.corp.sgi.com with the message *subscribe di-support <your e-mail address>* in the body (not the subject line) of your e-mail.

Fortility
The Over-40 infertility list can be reached via
http://www.surrogacy.com/fortility
Visit the web site to fill in an online subscription form, or send an e-mail with the message *subscribe* in the message body to: fortility-request@columbia.edu

i-List
An infertility e-mail group which offers a forum for dealing with infertility
through emotional support and exchange of information. To subscribe to
this mailing list, send an e-mail to Majordomo@plusnet.org with the
following command in the body (not the subject line) of your e-mail
message: *subscribe ilist*

Klinefelter's
There are two e-mail support groups for men with Klinefelter's syndrome
available through ONElist: SCA (Sex Chromosome Anomaly) and The
xxynetwork. See http://www.onelist.com for details on how to subscribe.

Miscarriage After Infertility
To subscribe to this list send an e-mail with the message *subscribe mai* in
the message body to: listserv@listserv.acsu.buffalo.edu

Mothers via Egg Donation
Visit the TASC website (http://www.surrogacy.com) to fill in an online
subscription form.

ONNA
This is an open discussion group, primarily made up of women who are
trying to conceive and who are finding that it takes longer than expected.
Subscribers are able to provide one another with information, shared
experiences and essential emotional support.
    To subscribe to the ONNA mailing list, visit the ONElist mailing list
site at: http://www.onelist.com/subscribe.cgi/onna

Pregnancy After Infertility
The purpose of this list, monitored by Valerie Singer, is to allow discussion of pregnancy concerns and experiences among people who have
struggled with infertility or recurrent miscarriage and have now achieved
pregnancy. Others with an interest, such as women who have already had
their 'infertility babies', are welcome to join in. To subscribe, send a
message to external-majordomo@palladium.corp.sgi.com with the message *subscribe panfert <your e-mail address>* in the body (not the subject
line) of your e-mail.

UK-Buddies Infertility List
Specifically for people in the UK to discuss all aspects of fertility treatments. To subscribe, visit:
http://www.onelist.com/subscribe.cgi/uk-buddies

Further Reading

FACTS AND HANDBOOKS

The HFEA publishes some very valuable information for anyone considering or undergoing infertility treatment. *The Patients' Guide to DI and IVF Clinics* (1997 edition) gives comprehensive details about the treatments carried out in each licensed clinic and the outcomes of those treatments. Lists of ICSI centres, sperm donor recruitment centres and egg donation centres are also available. A useful leaflet, *Treatment Clinics: Questions to Ask*, is also available. The annual HFEA reports also provide interesting information about recent developments, ethical concerns and research projects currently licensed. In addition, the HFEA *Code of Practice* will provide useful information for anyone considering or undergoing treatment at an HFEA-licensed clinic.

ISSUE, too, has produced a guide to all the clinics in the UK which offer various treatments for infertility. It gives information on whether they accept NHS patients, the investigations and treatments they carry out, whether there are any restrictions on whom they will treat (age limits, for example), waiting times and the costs of treatment. The booklet is free to members of ISSUE, or available for £1.50 from: Issue, 114 Lichfield Street, Walsall, WS1 1SZ.

FURSE, Anna, *The Infertility Companion*, Thorson's, 1997
Provides a comprehensive overview of the tests and options available, in the context of the social and economic parameters that will determine your chances of treatment. Also contains a very useful summary of treatment centres in the UK and the facilities they offer to help you make an informed choice. A good account of IVF treatment from someone who has experienced it herself, with the aim of making people undergoing tests and treatment feel more in control of the whole process.

JANSEN, Robert, *Overcoming Infertility: A Compassionate Resource to Getting Pregnant*, W.H. Freeman, 1997
A full and informative book on many aspects of infertility, which puts many myths and legends to rest.

NEUBERG, Roger, *Infertility: Tests, Treatment, Options*, Thorson's, 1991
A clinical guide to infertility and its investigations, from a consultant working in the field.

WINSTON, Robert, *Infertility: A Sympathetic Approach*, Optima, 1994
Written from the medical perspective of one of the most famous UK infertility experts, this book gives details about the tests and treatments available, along with your chances of success, in a straightforward, accessible way.

HELPING YOURSELVES

BARNES, Belinda and Suzanne Gail Bradley, *Planning for a Healthy Baby: Essential Reading for All Future Parents*. Ebury, 1995
All the recommendations of Foresight – the association for the promotion of preconceptual care – to do with diet, toxins, smoking and alcohol to maximise your chances of conception.

BERRYMAN, Julia, Karen Thorpe and Kate Windridge, *Older Mothers: Conception, Pregnancy and Birth after 35*, Pandora, 1995
Informative reading for any woman over 35 who has decided to try for a baby, including information about fertility rates and risks, and 'case histories' of first-time mid-thirties' mothers.

CLUBB, Elizabeth and Jane Knight, *Fertility: Fertility Awareness and Natural Family Planning*, David & Charles, 1996
While the emphasis is on ways of avoiding conception, the detailed information about interpreting BBT charts and cervical mucus changes (especially in particular situations such as just after coming off the contraceptive pill or if menopause is approaching) may help couples who are keeping track of their own cycles.

WESSON, Nicky, *Alternative Infertility Treatments: Enhance Your Optimum Health and Improve Your Chances of Conceiving*, Vermilion, 1997
Looks at natural ways of improving your chances of conception, including a range of alternative treatments from acupuncture to reflexology, as well

as discussing lifestyle changes you can make, including diet, relaxation techniques and exercise.

WHITWORTH, Belinda, *The Natural Way with Infertility: A Comprehensive Guide to Effective Treatment*, Element, 1996
Describes a range of therapies and discusses the benefits each could bring to solving fertility problems.

Two information booklets produced by the Department of Health, *Folic Acid and the Prevention of Neural Tube Defects*, and *While You Are Pregnant: Safe Eating and How to Avoid Infection from Food and Animals*, are available from: The Department of Health, Health Publications Unit, Heywood Stores, No. 2 Site, Manchester Road, Heywood, OL10 2PZ.

ENDOMETRIOSIS

HAWKRIDGE, Caroline, *Living with Endometriosis*, Vermilion, 1996
An informative book that summarises current thinking on endo, its causes and treatments. Getting the endo accurately diagnosed is a major problem for many women and the book looks at this aspect, together with offering suggestions for managing the pain and discussing the various treatments – hormonal, surgical and alternative therapies – and the subjects of infertility, pregnancy, and the emotional impact that endo can have on a woman's life.

MEARS, Jo, *Coping with Endometriosis*, Sheldon, 1997
A guide, endorsed by the National Endometriosis Society, to the causes, symptoms and treatments of this disease. The inclusion of case studies aims to help women analyse and understand their symptoms in an informed way, so as to be better prepared to talk to health professionals and to make the right choices for a treatment that suits them.

The National Endometriosis Society (address on p 279) provides a wide range of publications and factsheets on various medical, surgical and hormonal treatments, as well as a quarterly newsletter, *Endolink*. Call 0171 222 2781 for details.

MALE INFERTILITY

MASON, Mary-Claire, *Male Infertility: Men Talking*, Routledge, 1993
Men talking openly and honestly about how they reacted to a diagnosis

that they were infertile, with accounts of their medical experiences and the effect it had on their relationships.

SNOWDEN, Robert and Elizabeth, *The Gift of a Child: A Guide to Donor Insemination*, Allen & Unwin, 1993
A clear guide to male infertility, including the experiences of families who opted to overcome the infertility of the male partner by choosing donor insemination.

More information about sperm donation is available in a leaflet, *Important Information for Semen Donors*, published by the Royal College of Obstetricians and Gynaecologists. This is available from the HFEA (for address see p. 278) Two leaflets, *Egg Donation* and *Sperm and Egg Donors and the Law*, are also available from the HFEA.

A picture book called *My Story* helps parents explain their original to children conceived by DI. It is available from the DI Network (for address see p. 283).

MISCARRIAGE AND PREGNANCY LOSS

KOHNER, Nancy and Alix Henley, *When a Baby Dies*, Thorson's, 1997
The experiences and stories of couples who have lost a baby through late miscarriage, stillbirth, or death shortly after birth.

MOULDER, Christine, *Miscarriage: Women's Experiences*, Pandora, 1995
Information and personal stories from women who have suffered one or more miscarriages.

RAAB, Diana, *Getting Pregnant and Staying Pregnant*, Piccadilly, 1993
Written by a nurse who herself experienced delayed conception and miscarriage, this is an informative book about infertility, pregnancy complications, tests and pregnancy loss.

REGAN, Lesley, *Miscarriage*, Bloomsbury, 1997
Professor Regan, drawing on her experience as Professor of Obstetrics and Gynaecology and running the Miscarriage Clinic at St Mary's Hospital, London, describes the facts, the traumas and the hopes for the future in a way that will help to alleviate the emotional pain of those who are grieving after a miscarriage and to give encouragement to those who want to become pregnant again.

SURROGACY

Changing Conceptions of Motherhood: The Practice of Surrogacy in Britain, British Medical Association, 1996.
The report on surrogacy which reversed the BMA's previous stance and declared it acceptable, stressing the benefits of both the intended parents and the surrogate supporting each other through the process. A booklet called: *Considering Surrogacy? Your Questions Answered,* issued by the BMA in conjunction with the HFEA, provides a practical guide for anyone thinking of this as an option.

ADOPTION

CARGREAVES, Kate, *Journey to Our Children,* Aurora, 1996
One couple's story of infertility and adoption.

CHENNELLS, Prue and Chris Hammond, *Adopting a Child: A Guide for People Interested in Adoption,* British Agencies for Adoption and Fostering, 1995
Practical information about adoption and fostering.

PARENTING AFTER INFERTILITY

LASKER, Judith and Susan Borg, *In Search of Parenthood,* Pandora, 1989
Drawing on interviews from the USA, this book gives a real picture of what it is like to undergo assisted conception treatment and how it feels to be a parent of high-tech (often multiple) children.

MOODY, Jane, Jane Britten and Karen Hogg, *Breastfeeding Your Baby,* NCT, 1996
A full discussion of the physiology and practicalities of breastfeeding, with much useful information about feeding multiples and premature babies, together with fact files to help you sort out any difficulties especially in the early days.

GLAZER, Ellen Sarasohn, *Long-Awaited Stork: A Guide to Parenting after Infertility,* Lexington Books, USA (available in UK through CHILD), 1994
For new parents who have experienced infertility and gone on to have a family either through natural or assisted conception, or through adoption and fostering. It deals directly with the emotional impact of trying to be the 'perfect parent' after having waited so long.

MARSHALL, Fiona, *Coping with Postnatal Depression: Why It Happens and How to Overcome It*, Sheldon, 1993
A practical and reassuring guide for those with the baby blues or more serious, long-term depression.

COMING TO TERMS WITH INFERTILITY

HOUGHTON, Diane and Peter, *Coping with Childlessness*, Unwin Hyman, 1987
Written by a couple who are themselves 'involuntarily childless', it discusses their own experiences and those of others in conjunction with their work at ISSUE.

AND FINALLY . . .

KENNEDY, Angus J., *The Rough Guide to the Internet and World Wide Web*, Rough Guides Limited/Penguin, 1998
A book that will explain to the uninitiated every step of the way from signing on with a service provider to accessing mailing lists.

Glossary

A GUIDE TO ACRONYMS

In infertility treatment, a great many abbreviations are used. Below are some of those you may come across frequently in your notes or in your reading. This list will help you to find the right term in the glossary which follows.

AIH Artificial insemination by husband
AID Artificial insemination by donor
ART Sometimes used to stand for 'Advanced Reproductive Technologies' and sometimes 'Assisted Reproduction Technologies'. In either case it refers to the whole spectrum of medical techniques used to help infertile couples
BBT Basal body temperature
CVS Chorionic villus sampling
D&C Dilatation and curettage
DI Donor insemination
DIPI Direct intraperitoneal insemination
DNA Deoxyribonucleic acid (the abbreviation is nearly always used)
ET Embryo transfer
FSH Follicle-stimulating hormone
GIFT Gamete intrafallopian transfer
GnRH Gonodotrophin-releasing hormone
HFEA Human Fertilisation and Embryology Authority
HPT Home pregnancy test
HRT Hormone replacement therapy
HSG Hysterosalpingogram
ICSI Intracytoplasmic sperm injection
IUI Intra-uterine insemination
IVF In vitro fertilisation

IUD Intra-uterine device
LH Luteinising hormone
LMP Last menstrual period
MESA Micro-epididymal sperm aspiration
OPK Ovulation predictor kit
PCOS Polycystic ovary syndrome
PCT Postcoital test
PESA Percutaneous epididymal sperm aspiration
PET Pre-embryo transfer
PGD Pre-implantation genetic diagnosis
RE Reproductive endocrinologist
SUZI Subzonal insertion
TESE Testicular sperm extraction
TSH Thyroid stimulating hormone
ZIFT Zygote intrafallopian transfer

A fuller list of acronyms and abbreviations used in infertility treatment, which covers some less common tests and procedures, is posted at http:// www. pinelandpress.com. There is also a glossary at:http://www.inciid.org/ glossary.html which may be helpful if you come across a new term.

DEFINITIONS

Abortion The term used by the medical profession for any pregnancy terminated before 24 weeks' gestation, whether this was induced or a natural miscarriage.

Adhesions Sometimes called adhesive tissue, these are bands of fibrous scar tissue which may form after an infection or surgery. Adhesions bind organs together in abnormal ways and can severely reduce fertility if they block, for example, the fallopian tubes.

Amenorrhoea Absence of periods. In primary amenorrhoea, periods never begin after puberty; in secondary amenorrhoea, a woman who has previously had periods, and who is not pregnant or breastfeeding, stops having them.

Amniocentesis In this diagnostic test, carried out around the 16th to 18th week of pregnancy, a small amount of the amniotic fluid that surrounds the baby in the womb is withdrawn via a needle using ultrasound guidance. Cells from this fluid can then be grown and examined for evidence of chromosomal abnormalities such as Down's syndrome, or neural tube defects such as spina bifida, in the developing foetus, though these results can take some weeks to be confirmed. Amniocentesis itself carries a risk (0.5–2 per cent) of causing a miscarriage.

Androgens The male sex hormones, responsible for the development of male characteristics such as a deep voice and facial hair. The principal androgen is testosterone.

Anovulation The absence of ovulation. This can happen as a result of an imbalance of hormones, and is also sometimes caused by other conditions such as extreme weight loss. An anovulatory cycle is a cycle in which ovulation does not occur.

Antibody If anything enters our bodies that our immune system considers 'foreign' – substances known in general as antigens – we produce antibodies. For example, if we are infected by a particular strain of bacteria, we will produce antibodies to fight that infection which will render the bacteria harmless. Antibodies are specific to the antigen they are created to fight, which is why levels of antibodies in the blood can show up if we are immune to a particular disease.

Artificial insemination The insertion of semen into a woman's cervix by a means other than sexual intercourse, usually by using a syringe, to help her conceive. There are two varieties of this technique used in infertility treatment: in artificial insemination by husband (AIH), the husband's (or partner's) sperm is used; in artificial insemination by donor (AID), the sperm will have been donated by someone not known to the couple.

Assisted conception Any procedure where there is medical intervention to help eggs and sperm get together for fertilisation.

Asthenozoospermia A condition in which fewer than 40 per cent of a man's sperm are 'motile' – swimming about in the way that they need to in order to journey through the woman's body to reach the egg.

Azoospermia If a man has this condition, it means that he is producing semen but it contains no sperm.

Basal body temperature (BBT) The temperature of the body in a normal, rested state. If a woman takes her temperature each morning (when she is at rest and before the activity of the day begins, which may cause fluctuations in temperature), she can put together a BBT chart. As the BBT rises slightly after ovulation, these charts can be used to help show when ovulation will occur and therefore predict when the optimum fertile time in each cycle will be.

Biopsy In a biopsy a surgeon removes a tiny sample of body tissue, such as from the endometrium, so that it can be analysed in a laboratory.

Biphasic A term used to refer to a BBT chart which shows a rise in temperature after ovulation.

Blastocyst An early embryo, consisting of many cells. The term is often used to refer to the embryo at the stage when it is ready to implant in the uterus.

Blighted ovum When a fertilised egg fails to develop into an embryo after implantation in the uterus, it is called a blighted ovum. It always results in miscarriage.

Buserelin The brand name of a drug commonly used during infertility treatment. It is given by nasal spray or injection and has the effect of temporarily suppressing ovulation by suppressing the pituitary and preventing the release of the egg.

Candida albicans This yeast-like infection, sometimes called thrush, can reduce fertility. It can affect the vagina, causing itching and discharge, and the penis, causing dryness. It is also sometimes found in the digestive tract and the mouth.

Capacitation A chemical alteration in the membrane of the head of the sperm, which must occur if the sperm is to penetrate the egg.

Cervical mucus The mucus produced in the cervical canal, which often becomes visible in the vagina. The mucus alters at different stages in the menstrual cycle under the influence of different hormones, thinning to an 'egg-white' consistency at around the time of ovulation, which allows easier passage of sperm into the woman's body.

Cervix The narrow entrance to the womb, sometimes called the cervical canal. The cervix can be felt at the top of the vagina.

Chlamydia An infection of the genito-urinary tract which can affect fertility, reducing the sperm count in men and, in women, sometimes leading to inflammation and damaged fallopian tubes.

Chorionic villus sampling A diagnostic test, usually carried out in early pregnancy, which involves taking a sample of the developing placental tissue (the chorion) and testing it for indications of genetic defects in the embryo. It carries a risk of miscarriage (2–4 per cent) and the results are not always clear, in which case amniocentesis may be offered to confirm the results.

Chromosome In humans, the DNA needed to provide the blueprint for the development of the body is organised into 23 pairs of chromosomes, making a total of 46. These 46 chromosomes are found in the nucleus of every cell of our bodies with the exception of the sex cells – the egg of a woman or the sperm of a man. Each egg and each sperm contains half the chromosomes needed to make a new human being, and it is when the two sets of chromosomes join at fertilisation that a unique genetic blueprint for a new person is formed.

Clinical pregnancy The stage of pregnancy at which an ultrasound scan reveals a foetal heart beating.

Clitoris The small bud of sensitive tissue at the front of the vulva where the labia join.

Clomid The brand name of a commonly used hormone, clomiphene citrate, which stimulates ovulation.

Coitus A technical term used to describe heterosexual intercourse in which ejaculation occurs in the vagina.

Colposcopy In this procedure a small telescope called a colposcope is used to examine the vagina and cervix, usually for the purpose of checking for abnormalities.

Combined factor infertility Infertility resulting from a disorder in both partners, not just one.

Conception The fertilisation of an egg by a sperm. 'Assisted conception' refers to the whole range of fertility treatments which help to bring an egg and a sperm together for fertilisation, either within or outside the body.

Congenital abnormality Any deformity or disease that a person is born with.

Contraception Sometimes called birth control, this is the use of various methods to prevent conception. These methods include pills containing hormones, condoms and IUDs, as well as 'natural' methods such as using BBT charts to avoid intercourse around the time of ovulation.

Corpus luteum The literal translation of this Latin term is 'yellow body'. It refers to the glandular tissue that develops in the follicle of an ovary after an egg has been released. The corpus luteum plays an active role in conception by releasing progesterone, which also supports early pregnancy, in the second or 'luteal' phase of the infertility cycle. It has a limited lifespan, so if pregnancy doesn't occur the corpus luteum begins to break down after about 14 days.

Cowper's glands Small glands in the male reproductive system which produce the lubricative pre-ejaculatory fluid.

Cryopreservation In fertility treatments, this term refers to the freezing of embryos or sperm in liquid nitrogen. Current technical capabilities do not allow eggs to be frozen and retrieved successfully.

Cyst An abnormal growth, usually benign (non-malignant, or non-cancerous), somewhere in the body. Cysts can be formed of liquid or semi-solid material but, if they can be felt, will feel like lumps.

Cytomegalovirus (CMV) CMV is one of the herpes group of viruses. It is very common; many people catch CMV at some time in their lives but most show only mild symptoms (such as a sore throat and swollen glands) and the virus is usually harmless. However, if a mother is infected for the first time during pregnancy, particularly in the first two trimesters, the virus can cause abnormalities in the unborn child, the severity of which will vary according to the extent of the infection at birth.

Cytoplasm The material between the nucleus of a cell and its surface.

Danazol A fertility drug often used in the treatment of endometriosis.

DES (Diethylstilboestrol) A hormone once given, mainly in the USA, to try to prevent miscarriage; it caused uterine abnormalities in some of the unborn girl babies.

Dilatation and curettage In a D&C the cervix is opened (dilatation) and the inside of the womb scraped (curettage). The procedure is sometimes done after a miscarriage to make sure there are no retained products of conception, and sometimes to take a sample of the endometrium.

Direct intraperitoneal insemination In DIPI, sperm are injected through the wall of the vagina into the abdominal cavity at around the time of ovulation. The procedure can only help women who are ovulating and whose fallopian tubes are open. If stimulation drugs have been taken, there is a risk of a multiple pregnancy.

Donor A person who donates something for the benefit of others. In the infertility field it refers to a man who donates sperm, a woman who donates eggs, or a couple who donate embryos for the use of other couples or for research.

Donor insemination The placing of donor sperm into a woman, usually at the cervical opening or in the cervical canal, to help her conceive.

Down's syndrome A range of disabilities caused by an extra chromosome in pair 21 (which is why this syndrome is sometimes called Trisomy 21). The chromosomal abnormality results in a person having learning difficulties and sometimes other medical problems, which may be mild or severe.

DNA The basic 'building block' of life, DNA contains all the information we need to grow and develop into the particular person we are. In humans, DNA forms 23 pairs of chromosomes. Certain parts of these chromosomes contain recognisable patterns that we call genes, which influence particular aspects of our development.

Dysmenorrhoea Painful menstruation.

Ectopic pregnancy This is a distressing condition in which the fertilised egg implants outside the uterus, most often in one of the fallopian tubes, although it can be elsewhere in the pelvic cavity. With no endometrium to nourish the egg, the pregnancy cannot develop normally. The growing embryo can damage the fallopian tube, and will have to be surgically removed. An ectopic can lead to a reduction in fertility, although pregnancy is still possible if the other tube remains open.

Egg Produced by the ovaries, this cell contains half the genetic information needed to make a new human being. It is sometimes also called an oocyte or an ovum (hence the term 'ovulation' for the release of an egg), or the 'female gamete'.

Egg collection The removal of eggs directly from a woman's ovaries, often done as part of IVF treatment. When a woman has received hormonal treatment to make her 'superovulate' (produce more than one egg), the eggs must be collected from the ovaries before they are released and lost in the body cavity. The eggs are sucked out of the ovaries using a needle (usually with ultrasound guidance), either through the abdomen or through the vaginal wall, under local or general anaesthetic. This procedure is sometimes also called 'oocyte aspiration'.

Egg donation A woman may give her own eggs for use by another couple. She will need hormonal treatment to make her produce several eggs, which are then retrieved through egg collection.

Ejaculate The seminal fluid, containing the sperm, which is released from a man's penis at the moment of orgasm.

Embryo This term is used to refer to the initial stages of development of an unborn child, from a fertilised egg until about eight weeks of gestation. After that, an embryo is considered to have developed into a foetus.

Embryo transfer The stage in IVF treatment when the embryos are placed into the woman's uterus using a catheter inserted through the vagina and cervix. Up to three embryos may be transferred according to current UK law. It is sometimes known as PET: pre-embryo transfer.

Endocrine glands The glands within the body that secrete hormones. Our bodies need hormones for all sorts of uses (for example, at times of shock the adrenal gland produces adrenalin in what is often called the 'fight or flight' response, which enables us to deal more effectively with potential danger). The endocrine glands in the pituitary, hypothalamus, ovaries and testicles produce hormones essential for successful reproduction, and these interact with each other in the endocrine system. An endocrinologist is a medical specialist in hormones.

Endometriosis A sometimes painful and debilitating condition in which the endometrial cells, which usually only line the walls of the uterus, grow elsewhere within the pelvis, often over the ovaries or fallopian tubes.

Endometrium The lining of the womb. This thickens during the menstrual cycle and, if an egg does not implant, is shed at menstruation (when you have your period). An endometrial biopsy is sometimes taken to check the cells lining the womb.

Epididymis The thin coiled tube in the testicles where sperm mature as they are carried towards the vas deferens.

Eugenics The idea of breeding 'better' babies through genetic manipulation.

Fallopian tube A fallopian tube leads from each ovary to the uterus. Each tube has filaments called fimbria which collect the egg after it has been released from the ovary, and the egg is then transported along the tube towards the uterus. At the same time, the tube can help to transport sperm in the opposite direction. It is within the outer end of the tube that conception often takes place. The tubes are sometimes surgically examined in a procedure known as a falloscopy.

Female factor Any reason why a woman might be infertile.

Ferning During your most fertile time, a smear of cervical mucus looked at through a microscope should look like ferns. A check on this 'ferning' effect is one of the tests you may come across in infertility treatment.

Fertile phase The number of days (approximately six) in each cycle in which intercourse may result in a pregnancy.

Fertility cycle A term sometimes used for the menstrual cycle.

Fertilisation A term sometimes used interchangeably with 'conception', to denote the moment when a sperm successfully penetrates an egg.

Fibroid Benign (non-malignant or non-cancerous) growths of fibrous tissue sometimes found in the muscular wall of the uterus. Sometimes they lead to complications with the implantation of an embryo and during pregnancy, but often they cause no problems at all.

Fimbria The open end of the fallopian tubes, which pick up the egg after ovulation.

Foetus A term used to describe an unborn child after the eighth week of pregnancy, when all the major organs are formed. Before eight weeks, the term 'embryo' is used.

Follicle Each ovary contains several hundred follicles, small sacs in which the eggs mature and develop. After ovulation, the emptied follicle produces the corpus luteum, which in turn produces progesterone.

Follicle-stimulating hormone (FSH) This hormone, produced in the pituitary, causes the eggs in the ovaries to ripen and stimulates the production of oestrogen. The hormone is also found in men, where it plays a part in the formation of sperm.

Gamete The basic contribution from each partner: a sperm or an egg.

Gamete intrafallopian transfer In this procedure, sperm and eggs (a maximum of three) are mixed outside the body and transferred to the woman's fallopian tubes. The aim is to make it easier for fertilisation to occur inside the body.

Gene A section of DNA on our chromosomes. Genes determine how our bodies will grow, function and develop. Specific genes influence a particular inherited characteristic such as eye colour or height.

Genetic Relating to inherited characteristics. A genetic disorder is caused when something goes wrong with the chromosomes in the early stages of embryo development, and the normal development of an individual is then disrupted. Most embryos which contain damaged chromosomes either don't implant or aren't carried to term and a miscarriage results. Sometimes, however, a person may be born with a genetic abnormality such as Down's syndrome.

Genetic screening Some couples know that any children they produce are at risk of inheriting a defective gene from one or both of the parents. In genetic screening, embryos produced through IVF treatment are checked for the presence or absence of the defective gene before they are transferred into the woman's body.

Genitals The external parts of the male or female reproductive system.

Genito-urinary tract In both men and women the reproductive and excretory systems are closely linked. For example, both urine and sperm are released from the man's body via the penis. The genito-urinary tract or system is a term used to describe the organs involved in both processes.

Gestation The process by which a fertilised egg develops into an embryo, a foetus and then a baby. Gestation may begin outside the body but must always be completed within the body.

Gonadotrophin-releasing hormone (GnRH) Produced in the hypothalamus, GnRH stimulates the pituitary to release the gonadotrophins (the collective name for FSH and LH, the hormones responsible for egg development and ovulation).

Gonadotrophins Hormones secreted by the pituitary – LH and FSH. Gonadotrophin-releasing hormone stimulates the pituitary to send these hormones out.

Gonads The main sex glands: the ovaries and the testicles.

Graafian follicle A mature follicle in the ovary.

Granulosa cells 'Helper' cells which cluster round the egg, providing nutrients and releasing oestrogen.

Gynaecologist A doctor who specialises in the female reproductive system.

Haemorrhage Bleeding that cannot easily be controlled.

HPT Home pregnancy test; these days often as sensitive as clinic tests.

Hormone Chemicals which are produced and secreted by glands within the body and then carried through the bloodstream for a wide variety of purposes. The hormones used in reproduction can also be manufactured and introduced into the bloodstream.

Hostile mucus A term that describes a condition where a woman's cervical mucus does not successfully allow her partner's sperm through her cervix.

Human chorionic gonadotrophin (hCG) A hormone produced by the chorion, the membrane that surrounds the developing embryo. It maintains the corpus luteum beyond its usual lifespan so that it can continue to produce oestrogen and progesterone until the placenta has developed enough to take over. It is produced from a very early stage in embryo development, so its presence in the bloodstream is one of the earliest indicators of pregnancy. It is also used in IVF treatment just before egg collection, where it may be called your 'midnight injection'.

Human Fertilisation and Embryology Authority Set up in 1990, this is the body in the UK responsible for monitoring and recommending legislation on all aspects of assisted reproduction and for licensing centres where specific fertility treatments can be carried out.

Human menopausal gonadotrophin (hMG) A hormone extracted from the urine of women who have gone through the menopause (hence the name) which is used in fertility treatment to stimulate the follicles. A common brand name is Pergonal.

Humegon The brand name of a drug containing FSH, commonly used in infertility treatment. Administered by injection, it stimulates egg maturation within the follicles of the ovary, and egg release.

Hyperstimulation A very strong response to drugs that stimulate the ovaries, sometimes causing the ovaries to swell and producing a range of side-effects.

Hypothalamus The part of the brain that controls the pituitary.

Hysterosalpingogram In this procedure, dye is pushed through a woman's uterus and fallopian tubes. An X-ray can then show up any blockages.

Hysteroscopy An inspection of the inside of the uterus using a small viewing scope.

Immotile Describes sperm that aren't swimming as they should be.

Implantation The stage when the fertilised egg embeds itself in the endometrium.

Intracytoplasmic sperm injection In ICSI, a single sperm is injected into an egg in the laboratory and returned to the woman's uterus after fertilisation. This technique is often used to help men with low sperm counts.

Intrauterine device An IUD is a form of contraception which works by preventing implantation of an embryo.

Intrauterine insemination In IUI, specially treated semen is injected through the woman's cervical canal into her uterus to increase the couple's chances of conceiving.

In vitro fertilisation Eggs are gathered from the woman's ovaries and mixed with sperm in a laboratory dish to achieve fertilisation outside the body. Up to three of the resulting embryos can be transferred to the woman's uterus.

Klinefelter's syndrome A chromosomal condition in which the man has an extra X chromosome, which usually results in sterility.

Laparoscopy A surgical procedure in which a small cut is made in the abdomen so that the internal organs can be viewed through a long, thin instrument with a light source, called a laparoscope. A laparoscopy is often used in infertility investigations as it allows the surgeon to check the condition of the ovaries and fallopian tubes.

Live birth The delivery of one or more babies from a pregnancy. In fertility treatments, the 'live birth rate' is calculated as a proportion of live births for every 100 treatment cycles started.

Luteal phase The part of the cycle after ovulation, in which the corpus luteum develops; it usually lasts about 14 days.

Luteal phase defect (LPD) There are two types of luteal phase defects: a short phase of about 10 days or less; or one which is not necessarily shorter than the standard 12–16 days, but progesterone production is low. Luteal phase problems can mean that this part of the cycle doesn't last long enough to allow an embryo to implant, often because the corpus luteum breaks down too quickly and menstruation begins.

Luteinising hormone A hormone secreted by the pituitary gland: rising LH levels trigger ovulation. In men, LH plays a role in stimulating the testes to produce testosterone.

Male factor Any reason why a man might be infertile.

Menarche The start of a woman's reproductive life, usually marked by the first menstrual period.

Menopause The end of the reproductive phase of a woman's life, when her periods gradually stop. A woman who has a premature menopause will find that her body loses its fertile capabilities much earlier than usual, perhaps in her twenties.

Menstrual cycle The fertility cycle of a woman's body, in which the female sex hormones work together to bring about physiological changes concerned with producing an egg and preparing the uterus for possible pregnancy or menstruation.

Menstruation A woman's 'periods'. The shedding of the endometrium from the uterus, normally about two weeks after ovulation, if the egg is not fertilised. While it is often called the 'monthly' period, the cycle may be more or less than 28 days.

Metrodin The brand name of a drug commonly used in infertility treatment. Administered by injection, it stimulates ovulation.

Micro-epididymal sperm aspiration (MESA) In this procedure sperm are extracted from the epididymis in a surgical operation and can then be used to fertilise an egg.

Micromanipulation Techniques used in IVF to get a sperm past the protein shell of the egg.

Microsurgery An operation in which the surgeon looks through special microscopes to carry out delicate and detailed work using precision instruments on very small parts of the body, such as the fallopian tubes.

Mid-cycle A term used to refer to the fertile phase, the days around which ovulation should occur, though for some women this won't be the precise mid-point of their cycle.

Miscarriage The spontaneous and complete loss of a developing embryo or foetus in the first 24 weeks of pregnancy. Medical staff often refer to a miscarriage as an abortion.

Monophasic A term used to refer to a BBT chart which shows no rise in temperature, indicating that ovulation is probably not occurring.

Mosaicism A condition in which the chromosomes of the body are not the same in every cell.

Motility A measurement of the movement capabilities of a man's sperm.

Multiple birth The birth of two or more babies from a single pregnancy. (A multiple birth is still a single 'live birth event' in HFEA figures.) If you are expecting twins or more, you're having a multiple pregnancy.

Neural tube defect A problem with the development of the brain or spinal cord. In one such defect, spina bifida, the spinal cord and vertebrae have not formed completely. Neural tube defects range in severity but can cause physical or mental disabilities.

Nuchal scan Using ultrasound, the nuchal fold at the back of the unborn baby's neck is measured. A wider than usual fold can indicate an increased chance of the baby having Down's syndrome.

Obstetrician A doctor who specialises in pregnancy and labour.

Oestradiol (E2) A hormone produced by the ovaries as the eggs mature.

Oestrogen A hormone, produced mainly by the ovaries, which governs female sexual development and fertility. Increasing levels of oestrogen in the pre-ovulation phase of the cycle affect the cervix, cervical mucus and endometrium.

Oligospermia A low number of sperm in the semen (less than 20 million per millilitre).

Oocyte An egg (the term is sometimes used to indicate an egg that is not yet mature).

Ovarian hyperstimulation syndrome A rare but serious reaction to drugs designed to stimulate the ovaries into producing many eggs.

Ovary A woman usually has two ovaries, one each side of her uterus, which contain the eggs, of which several will ripen in each menstrual

cycle. The ovaries also produce the hormones oestrogen and progesterone.

Ovulation The release of a mature egg (ovum) from one of the follicles in
the ovaries.

Ovulation predictor kit OPKs, which can be used at home, measure the
presence of luteinising hormone in the urine. As the LH surge triggers
ovulation each month, they can be used to help time intercourse so that
it coincides with the most fertile phase of the cycle.

Ovum The mature sex cell containing the mother's genes produced by
the ovaries (also called a gamete, but more usually an egg). The plural is
ova.

Patency A term you may hear which simply indicates that everything is
open and working in your reproductive system.

Pelvic inflammatory disease Any infection which affects the female
reproductive organs, which can result in scarring and adhesions which
cause infertility.

Penis One of the external male reproductive organs. The urethra which
runs through the penis carries urine from the bladder and semen
(containing sperm from the testes).

Percutaneous epididymal sperm aspiration Taking sperm directly from
the epididymis via a hollow needle (PESA) introduced through the
skin. The sperm can then be used to fertilise an egg.

Pergonal The brand name of a drug commonly used in infertility treatment.
Administered by injection, it contains FSH and LH which stimulate egg
maturation within the follicles of the ovary, and egg release.

Perinatal death Sometimes called a stillbirth, this is the loss of a baby
after 24 weeks of pregnancy or just after birth.

Pituitary A gland at the base of the brain which produces many hormones, including FSH and LH, which control the ovaries and testes and
trigger them into making their own hormones.

Polycystic ovary syndrome Women with PCOS have many small, follicular cysts on their ovaries, which can prevent ovulation. PCOS is the
most common endocrine disorder, affecting approximately 6 per cent
of premenopausal women. It's also associated with other distressing
side-effects such as weight gain, irregular periods, acne and excessive
body hair growth, depending on its severity.

Polyps Small benign growths, smaller than fibroids, in the uterus.

Postcoital test The investigation of cervical mucus after intercourse
(around the time of ovulation) to check for the presence of sperm,
and whether they are likely to get through to fertilise the egg.

Preconceptual care Making sure you're both in optimum health before
conceiving.

Pre-eclampsia A condition of pregnancy marked by high blood pressure, protein in the urine and oedema (fluid retention and swelling in the limbs). It can pose a severe threat to the health of both mother and baby, which may necessitate induction or an emergency caesarean before eclampsia (convulsions and fits) develops. The condition always disappears after delivery.

Pre-embryo A more precise term used to describe an embryo up until about 14 days of development, or when the 'primitive streak' develops, which is the first sign that the cells are beginning to differentiate. No research may be done on an embryo after this point.

Pregnancy The gestation of a baby in a woman's womb until birth. In a 'clinical pregnancy' there are signs of a foetal heart beating at about seven weeks, though not all clinical pregnancies go on to become live births. A positive pregnancy test that is followed by menstruation can indicate that implantation of an embryo did occur, but that hormone levels weren't high enough to ensure that the pregnancy continued.

Pre-implantation genetic diagnosis A technique which screens an in vitro embryo for genetic abnormalities. One or two cells are removed from the embryo while it is still in vitro and these are tested to determine the sex of the embryo and its genetic make-up, usually to check for an inherited disorder.

Pre-ovulation phase The first part of the fertility cycle, from the onset of menstruation to ovulation, which may vary considerably in length.

Primary infertility Being infertile when you have never had a pregnancy.

Progesterone A hormone produced by the corpus luteum in the ovary after ovulation. It prepares the endometrium for pregnancy and, as its levels increase in the bloodstream, the body's basal temperature rises.

Prolactin A hormone produced by the pituitary in both men and women. Its main effect is to stimulate the production of breastmilk but it also inhibits the ovaries from producing oestrogen, which is why high levels of prolactin in the bloodstream can interfere with fertility.

Prostate A gland situated just beneath the bladder in men. It secretes nutrients into the seminal fluid.

Provera A form of progesterone, given either through tablets or as an injection.

Puberty The time in our lives when our secondary sexual characteristics develop under the influence of increasing levels of hormones, and our reproductive systems start to function.

Reproductive endocrinologist A medical specialist in the endocrine system and the hormones produced by the body for successful reproduction.

Salpingitis Infection and inflammation of the fallopian tubes.

Salpingogram An X-ray of the fallopian tubes

Salpingostomy An operation to open or repair (salpingoplasty) a blocked fallopian tube.

Secondary infertility The condition in which you have had a pregnancy (though not necessarily a baby) but can't conceive again.

Secondary sexual characteristics The features that develop at puberty which are particular to our sex. Boys, influenced by androgens, will gradually develop deeper voices and beards, for example, while girls, influenced by oestrogen, will develop breasts.

Selective reduction The deliberate abortion of one of more foetuses in a multiple pregnancy to give the remaining ones a better chance of survival.

Semen (seminal fluid) The fluid ejaculated from the penis during orgasm. It is made up of secretions from the seminal vesicles and the prostate, and it may or may not contain sperm.

Semen analysis A test sometimes called a 'sperm count', to check the semen for volume, sperm density, motility, forward progression, morphology (the sperm should have an oval head and a long tail), whether there is any sperm 'clumping' or any thickening of the seminal fluid, and whether there are high levels of white or red blood cells present.

Seminal vesicles Two sacs in the male reproductive tract which secrete part of the seminal fluid into the urethra.

Seminiferous tubules The long tubes in the testicles where sperm develop.

Sexually transmitted disease Any infection that is transmitted from one person to another through sexual contact.

Sperm Sometimes called spermatozoon, plural spermatozoa, a sperm is a mature male sex cell containing the father's genes. An immature sperm is called a spermatid.

Spermicide A substance that kills sperm (as is found, for instance, in spermicidal condoms).

Spinnbarkeit A term used to describe the stretchiness or elasticity which characterises 'fertile' cervical mucus, the sort that allows the easy passage of sperm.

Spotting Small amounts of blood or brownish discharge which occur during the fertility cycle at times outside a true period.

Standardised selective salpingography In conjunction with an HSG, a catheter is passed through the cervix and into the opening of the fallopian tube. Dye is then squirted along the tube at high pressure, which can clear any blockages. This procedure can be a preferred option to surgery to try to unblock fallopian tubes as it requires no general anaesthetic.

Sterile Someone who is permanently and completely infertile, rather than just 'subfertile', where conception may be delayed but is not impossible.

Subzonal insemination In this technique (SUZI), a single sperm is injected into the egg just beneath the zona pellucida.

Superovulation A process in which a woman's ovaries are stimulated with fertility hormones to produce many eggs.

Surrogate mother A woman who bears a child for someone else. In straight surrogacy, the surrogate provides the egg; in host surrogacy, IVF will provide an embryo that can be implanted into the surrogate.

Swim-up test A test to check the percentage of abnormal sperm a man produces, or to separate out the normal sperm which are then used for insemination.

Tamoxifen The brand name of a drug commonly used in infertility treatment, which mimics the effects of oestrogen and stimulates ovulation.

Temperature chart See BBT chart.

Testes The testicles (singular, testis). The two male glands which produce sperm and the sex hormones, including testosterone.

Testicular sperm extraction In this procedure (TESE) sperm are removed directly from the testicles.

Testosterone The principal male sex hormone, produced in the testes. Small amounts of testosterone are also produced in women.

Thyroid-stimulating hormone This is occasionally used in fertility treatment if one of the couple is suspected of having an underactive thyroid gland.

Toxoplasmosis This infection is caused by a parasite found in cat faeces, raw meat and contaminated soil. It causes few symptoms in a healthy adult, who may not even be aware of the infection, but can have serious effects on an unborn child, including brain damage and blindness. Many pregnant women will already be immune and immunity can be screened for antenatally. Precautions for pregnant women, or for those hoping to conceive, include: always wear gloves when gardening; wash all fruit and vegetables; wash your hands after handling raw meat; get someone else to empty the cat-litter tray.

Triple test One of several blood screening tests which may be offered in early pregnancy to help assess the risk of having a baby with Down's syndrome or neural tube defects such as spina bifida. It measures the level of three substances in the blood: alphafetoprotein, unconjugated oestriol and human chorionic gonadotrophin. Other, similar, blood screening tests include the double test, the multimarker test, triple-plus test and Bart's test.

Tubal insufflation A test, rarely used these days, to check whether the fallopian tubes are open by blowing gas through them.

Turner's syndrome A chromosomal condition affecting women in which the sex chromosome is completely absent in all the body's cells meaning that she is completely infertile. Sometimes there is a mosaicism, which can reduce fertility.

Ultrasound A diagnostic technique in which high-frequency sound waves (rather than X-rays) are used to produce an image of what's happening inside the body. It can be done by moving a transducer across the abdomen, or vaginally.

Undescended testes A condition in which one or both of the testes stays in the abdomen rather than moving down into the scrotum, which can result in permanent damage to sperm production.

Urethra The name of the tube (in both men and women) along which urine is expelled from the body. In men the urethra, which runs through the penis, also carries semen.

Uterus The womb. It is in the uterus that the unborn child develops throughout pregnancy. Pregnancy begins when a fertilised egg successfully implants in the lining of the uterus (the endometrium). A 'retroverted' uterus is one that is tilted slightly backwards.

Vagina The canal that leads from the cervix of the uterus to the opening in a woman's vulva.

Varicocoele A swollen vein around the testes (sometimes called a varicole).

Vas deferens The tube from each testicle which carries the semen to the urethra.

Vasectomy An operation in which the vas deferens in each testicle is surgically closed in order to sterilise a man.

Vasogram Dye is injected into the vas deferens and an X-ray taken which will show up any blockages that might be preventing the sperm from reaching the semen.

Vulva The external female genitals – the labia and clitoris.

Zoladex The brand name of a drug commonly used during infertility treatment. It's given by nasal spray or injection and has the effect of temporarily suppressing ovulation.

Zona pellucida The outer layer of an egg which a sperm has to penetrate in order to fertilise the egg.

Zygote The single cell that results when an egg and a sperm fuse. After further cell division, the zygote is called an embryo.

Zygote intrafallopian transfer ZIFT is similar to GIFT except that the sperm and eggs are mixed outside the body and it is the resulting fertilised egg (rather than the gametes) which is then transferred to the fallopian tubes while the woman is under general anaesthetic.

Index

and embryo freezing 140, 142
and failure 258
and IVF 98, 115
legal requirements xiv, 98
organisations 282
and surrogacy 171, 173, 177,
190
Cowper's glands 12, 313
cremasteric muscles 11
crossover test 68
cryopreservation, see embryo,
frozen
cystic fibrosis xii, 135, 148–9,
173
cysts 313
ovarian 58, 66, 69, 72, 73,
106, 108, 143

D&C 74, 314
depression 258
DES (diethylstilboestrol) 198,
314
diabetes 16, 55, 61, 68, 170, 299
diagnosis, coming to terms with
80–2
diet 22, 24, 41, 272
dieting 24
disability xii, 50, 85–6, 88, 111,
174
disclosure 218–20
discontinuing treatment 260–3
doctor, see GP
donation xiii, 145–66
considering 149–50
donor 147–9, 164–5, 314
egg donation 78, 79, 80, 98,
155, 157–63
emotional aspects 228
legal aspects 146–7, 151, 155,
164
matching recipient and donor
149

organisations 282–3
screening 148–9
donor insemination (DI) 79, 80,
145–6, 150–3, 314
considering 149–50
information sources 301
Down's syndrome 157, 244, 314
drugs xiii, 12, 61, 170
see also hormone treatment;
medication
Duchenne's muscular dystrophy
135, 145

e-mail 232–4
ectopic pregnancy 59, 129, 314
information sources 300
previous 137, 203
recognising 236
and smoking 29
treatment 195–6
and tubal surgery 109
egg 4–5, 314
collection 122–4, 139, 147,
154, 315
cultivation 117–19
frozen 148
implantation 5, 7
lifespan 26
maturation 58
release of 4–5, 6, 13
tests 73
egg donation 157–63, 315
donors 147–8, 153–7, 160–1,
163
information sources 277, 302
in IVF 78, 98
in surrogacy 79
unexplained infertility 80
waiting time 155
ejaculation 12, 146, 315
embryo 315
choosing 127–8

A NOTE ON THE AUTHOR

Anna McGrail is a writer and editor in the
field of health and social care, and a regular
contributor to parenting magazines. She is
the author of *You and Your New Baby*,
which won an award from the British
Medical Association, and *Crying*, a practical
handbook for coping with crying babies.